Handbook for Hospital Ethics Committees

by Judith Wilson Ross
with Sister Corrine Bayley, Vicki Michel, and Deborah Pugh

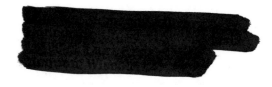

American Hospital Publishing, Inc.,
a wholly owned subsidiary of the
American Hospital Association

Library of Congress Cataloging in Publication Data

Ross, Judith Wilson.
    Handbook for hospital ethics committees.

    "Catalog no. 025101" — T.p. verso.
    Bibliography: p.
    Includes index.
    1. Medical ethics. 2. Hospital care — Moral and
ethical aspects. 3. Ethics committees. I. Title.
[DNLM: 1. Ethics. 2. Hospitals. 3. Professional
Staff Committees. WX 159 R824h]
R725.3.R67 1986   174'.2   86-14130
ISBN 0-939450-96-8

Catalog no. 025101

Text sets in Times Roman
3M—3/86—0149
2.5M—3/88—0210
2M—8/89—0247
1M—11/90—0287
2M—2/91—0293
2M—5/92—0320

Audrey Kaufman, Editor
Peggy DuMais, Production Coordinator
Brian Schenk, Acquisitions and Editorial Manager
Dorothy Saxner, Vice-President, Books

Table of Contents

About the Authors

Judith Wilson Ross, M.A., is an associate at the Center for Bioethics, St. Joseph Health System (Orange, CA) and associate director of the University of California-Los Angeles Program in Medical Ethics. She teaches and writes about medical ethics and is the coauthor of *The Insanity Plea* (1983) and *Choosing Life or Death: A Guide for Patients, Families, and Professionals* (1986).

Sister Corrine Bayley, M.A., is a vice-president at St. Joseph Health System (Orange, CA), and director of its Center for Bioethics. She is nationally known as a writer and lecturer on bioethics and the role of hospital ethics committees and has been instrumental in the creation and development of ethics committees throughout the country.

Vicki Michel, M.A., J.D., is associate professor at Loyola School of Law (Los Angeles), where she teaches law, including legal and ethical issues in health care. She also chairs the Los Angeles County Bar Association's Bioethics Committee and is a member of the Los Angeles County Bar Association and Medical Association Joint Committee on Biomedical Ethics.

Deborah Pugh, R.N., M.N., is a nurse-ethicist and is director of the Center for Human Development, St. Joseph Health System (Orange, CA). She has been a consultant to many ethics committees and is a frequent lecturer on bioethics.

Preface

Over the past few years, the Center for Bioethics, St. Joseph Health System (Orange, CA), has received many queries and requests for information about the nature and operation of ethics committees. We are grateful to all those who called or wrote letters, because their questions encouraged us to think more deeply about how ethics committees should and could function.

This book is first a formal response to those queries: an attempt to answer the questions in a systematic fashion. Second, it is an attempt to provide the knowledge gathered from ethics committees that have pioneered this work to ethics committees that are just starting out and to people who are just beginning to serve on such committees. Finally, we hope this book will provide a second generation of questions for ethics committees that have by now come to terms with the first generation of questions.

We extend our sincere thanks to all the ethics committee members who have so generously shared their experiences with us. Without their work, this book would not have been possible. We wish, as well, to acknowledge the support of the California Association of Catholic Hospitals, which made the initial writing of this book possible. Finally, we want to thank those who read and commented on the manuscript: William J. Winslade, Ph.D., J.D., Institute of Medical Humanities, Galveston, Texas; Cheryl Steffen, L.C.S.W., chairman, Bioethics Committee, St. Joseph Hospital, Orange, California; Evelyn Van Allen, coordinator, Minnesota Network for Institutional Ethics Committees; Elliot Dorff, Ph.D., provost, University of Judaism, Los Angeles, California; Reverend Jeremiah McCarthy, St. John's Seminary, Camarillo, California; Mary L. Ahern, assistant general counsel, American Hospital Association; and several anonymous readers. They gave us criticism that was always helpful, in a manner that was always gracious.

This book is not a definitive statement on the role of ethics committees in health care. It is an initial statement of where we find ourselves now and what our experiences have been so far. We do not know the future of ethics committees. That will depend, at least in part, on the quality of care that ethics committee members put into their work. What we *do* know is that the need to carefully consider ethical problems in patient care will continue to grow in the years to come.

Judith Wilson Ross
Sister Corrine Bayley
Vicki Michel
Deborah Pugh

Introduction

The ethical dilemmas of modern health care are, for the most part, a result of new technology, increased costs, cultural emphasis on individual rights, uncertain or conflicting social values, and changing relationships among health care professionals. Because the hospital has been dramatically changed by these forces in the past 20 years, traditional ways of handling problems are no longer adequate. Medical questions require medical answers, but many of the most puzzling questions that health care workers currently face are not exclusively medical in nature. They are questions about individual values, about the personal meaning of life and death, and about fairness and justice. Patients, doctors, nurses, social workers, religious advisers, hospital administrators, and society itself all need to take part in asking those questions and making those decisions, which not only affect individual lives but also shape social relations. Ethics committees represent an important response to that need for a broader range of thinking about critical health care decisions.

The creation of ethics committees provides an opportunity for health care providers as a group to grapple with hard questions and, thereby, to be able to understand and to respond better to the concerns of patients and society. Discussing ethical issues more openly and more frequently can lead not only to better decisions but also to better relationships among health care professionals. By probing ethical concerns together, ethics committee members can learn from one another and can learn to respect one another.

The brief experience of hospitals with ethics committees suggests that each institution will handle things a little differently; each will create a form that fits its own situation. There are, however, some common threads. First, the process of getting a committee functioning is slow. It may take a long time for the members to feel as if they are accomplishing something or are having any effect on institutional attitudes and behavior. That may be discouraging. Committees with extensive experience report that it takes a year or two before the members see or sense results of their work. Patience, compassion, and optimism are necessary virtues for ethics committee members. It also helps if the members work hard at listening carefully to one another with an openness to learning.

Second, committees may become bogged down in decisions about committee structure, rules, and procedural operations. Voting procedures, the number of people needed for a consultation, the type of minutes kept, and attendance requirements are concrete issues, amenable to fixed resolution. They are familiar kinds of issues and everyone is comfortable with his or her own opinion on these matters. The easiness of these issues can be unfortunate, for committees may fall into discussing these concrete matters rather than struggling through uncomfortable discussions about ethical issues. Agreeing on the principles that should guide decisions to forego treatment is much less concrete, much more likely to reveal conflict, and much more difficult than agreeing about who should be an ethics committee member or how long committee members should serve. Especially in their early stages, ethics committees need to be flexible about how they deal with procedural issues. A committee can successfully exist for a long time without making any of these nuts-and-bolts decisions. If committees do not commit themselves early to procedural discussions and decisions, they will have more time to do the hard work: educating themselves and discussing the ethical issues. In any case, ethics committees are far too new for anyone to know which procedures are "right" or "best." Decisions about procedures are likely to take care of themselves, once experience shows how the committee best functions within the institution.

Finally, the third common thread is that the committee will periodically struggle with its purpose, functions, and accountability. This is a natural, though frustrating, evolutionary process. However, one thing is certain, and committee members would do well to keep it in mind: *ethics committees should exist primarily to serve patients and to protect their interests.* The temptation to protect the hospital, hospital employees, and physicians will be felt frequently. In many situations, the interests of hospital, health care workers, and patients and families will be united; in other situations the patients' interests may appear obscure or uncertain; in yet others, the patients' preferences may lie in sharp contrast with the values of the hospital or of the health care professionals. It will be difficult to always keep the patients' interests uppermost and, in some cases, it will be impossible. If it were easy, ethics committees would not be needed. They are a potential solution to a problem: the problem is hard, and the solution is new. Ethics committee members should feel very unsure about the wisdom of their decisions, for they are walking on uncertain ground. If they can tolerate the perpetual ambiguity, they will find the results almost certainly rewarding.

This manual has been written to help committees through the initial period of uncertainty. It is, however, only an introduction to their work and may sometimes seem to be a very ambiguous guide. At its best, it is like those world maps of the medieval mapmakers, who were obliged to label large areas *terra incognita* but could helpfully point to other areas in which they knew "Here, there be dragons." This manual will point out several dragon-dwelling locales, some major historical monuments, a number of scenic views and points of interest, some well-traveled roads (as well as paths where the grass is scarcely beaten down), and some genuine *terra incognita.* It will not tell readers where to start or where to go. On this map there are many places to start, many possible destinations, and many routes. We have tried to provide the necessary background information, an initial discussion about ethics and the ethical principles that members need to know, some practical suggestions about administrative matters, an introduction to law and bioethics, and some examples of the work of ethics committees. Some sections will be helpful for educating new committee members; other parts can be referred to when the committee faces a specific problem.

In general, we see this manual as a work that committee members will refer to when they need information about a specific issue, rather than as a book that they will sit down with and read from cover to cover. Because of this, certain portions overlap. For example, although chapter 11 addresses privacy and confidentiality as separate topics, the issues flowing from an obligation to respect privacy and to ensure confidentiality are also discussed as one aspect of other topics, including case review in chapter 8, keeping records in chapter 7, and "Committee Liability," chapter 13. Where discussions are substantial, we have tried to provide cross-references in the text. However, readers should also refer to the index.

We hope that those committee members who stay with this journey will let us know where they have gone and what they found there. It will help us to make a more accurate map, and it will lead to more efficient, if less adventurous, journeys for those who come later.

Part I

Ethics and Health Care

Chapter 1

History of the Bioethics Movement

The 1954 Supreme Court decision in *Brown v. Board of Education* (the case in which school segregation was found unconstitutional) signalled a profound change in American society. The underlying message of that decision was embodied in the principle "respect for persons." Although the civil rights movement began with racial concerns, the insistence that individuals deserve respect as human beings quickly spread to demands for civil rights protection for other vulnerable groups: mental patients, women, children, and, eventually, medical patients. The doctrine of informed consent for medical care, although legally rooted in common law tort doctrine and constitutional privacy rights, is deeply indebted to the spirit of the times, which emphasized respect for persons and gave an unparalleled endorsement to individualism and individual rights.

Also born of this dominating concern for individual rights was the bioethics movement. In the mid-1960s and the early 1970s, a number of distinct issues and technological advances emerged—the discovery of ethically questionable medical research practices, the initial successes of organ transplantation, the development of long-term hemodialysis, the abortion reform movement, the use of ventilators with permanently unconscious patients, and the consumer-rights and patient-rights movements—all of which provided important impetus for the creation of the transdisciplinary field known as bioethics.

Medical Research

Extensive publicity about three research projects resulted in the establishment of the National Commission for the Protection of Human Subjects of Biomedical and Behavioral Research. The first project occurred in 1963, at the Jewish Chronic Disease Hospital (Brooklyn). Elderly patients with chronic illness were injected with live cancer cells in an effort to discover whether the cells would survive in a person who was ill but did not have cancer. The researchers had reason to believe the cells would not survive, but they did not obtain consent from patients or family members before proceeding. Although the responsible researchers had their licenses suspended, the suspension was stayed and they were placed on probation.

In the second research project, the U.S. Public Health Service conducted a study of poor, uneducated black men with syphilis in Tuskegee, Alabama, from 1932 to 1972. In the 1940s, penicillin became available for treating syphilis. Nevertheless, the researchers did not tell the subjects that treatment was available, nor did they provide it for them. Although objections to the study had been made in 1965, it was not until 1972, when information about the study became more widely publicized, that the Department of Health, Education and Welfare (DHEW) appointed a task force to assess what had gone wrong. The task force concluded that the study was "ethically unjustified" from the very beginning.

Finally, in 1967, mentally retarded children at the Willowbrook State School, New York, were given hepatitis by injection in a study that hoped to find a way to reduce the damage done by the disease. Hepatitis was endemic in most institutions, and researchers believed that all residents were likely to contract the disease eventually. Although consent was obtained in this study, the consent sometimes had an element of coercion, as it was difficult to gain placement in the institution and if parents consented to research participation the children were admitted both to the project and to the institution. Many critics questioned the morality of placing these extremely vulnerable children at additional risk.

In response to these events (especially the Tuskegee research), the National Commission for the Protection of Human Subjects was created in 1974 by public law. It worked through 1978 and by 1979 had published a series of reports and recommendations that were quickly incorporated into federal law. In addition, in 1979 the commission published *The Belmont Report: Ethical Principles and Guidelines for the Protection of Human Subjects of Research*. The most visible effect of the national commission was its recommendation that all institutions receiving research funds from the federal government establish an institutional review board (IRB). IRBs, which include both researchers and lay persons, serve to review all biomedical and behavioral research proposals to ensure that they meet ethical standards for protecting the rights of the potential subjects.[1]

The commission included researchers, but was made up primarily of individuals who approached the question of protecting human subjects from the perspective of law, philosophy, theology, history, and the social sciences. For many of these people, this was their first entry into ethical problems of research and medical practice: what later came to be called bioethics.

Organ Transplantation

In 1967, Christiaan Barnard first transplanted the human heart. In 1968, the Harvard Medical School ad hoc committee published its report, delineating brain-death criteria for use in pronouncing death in patients who were being maintained on respirators so that their organs could be used for transplantation.[2] The Harvard report led to the passage of brain-death statutes in many states. Such statutes were necessary because physicians risked being prosecuted for murder in organ donor situations. When all brain activity ceased, physicians wanted to remove the needed organs, even though the donor's heart and lungs continued to function with the support of the ventilator. Because heart-lung function continued, the donor was still legally alive if death could not be pronounced by brain-death criteria.

In addition to generating legislation, the success of heart as well as kidney transplantation encouraged extensive discussion about how enough donated organs could be acquired. As a result of this policy debate, the Uniform Anatomical Gift Act was adopted in many states. It seemed a relatively simple and obvious solution to the problem of authorizing donation, but, like many simple and obvious solutions, it has not worked. Although people say they favor donation, they rarely, in fact, complete the cards and, even when they do, hospitals frequently do not honor them. Despite the failure of the donor program, the debates about obtaining organ donations and about the acceptability of brain-death were important steps in bringing the bioethics movement to life.

Hemodialysis

Between 1960 (when long-term dialysis first became possible) and 1972 (when the federal government amended the Social Security Act to include medical coverage for all victims of end-stage renal disease), the first significant contemporary discussions about allocation of scarce resources were conducted. The artificial kidney was the first life-prolonging, high-technology treatment to capture the public's attention. As a result, many articles appeared discussing how to choose patients for dialysis treatment and whether or not everyone who needed dialysis was morally entitled to it. More than research or heart transplants, hemodialysis increased public interest in the ethical dimension of health care problems. In general, the public had responded to transplantation with awe at the achievements of science but had not perceived the ethical problems that were emerging. Research abuses also failed to present to the public clear ethical conflicts. The Tuskegee case or the Jewish Chronic Disease Hospital case had seemed, for the most part, plain wrong to most lay persons. However, shortages of dialysis equipment made the ethical dilemma both obvious and poignant. Specific individuals, some of whom appeared on television, were dying for lack of a treatment that was known and available—but not available to them.

The Synthesis: Bioethics

The field of bioethics came into existence because there was a need to talk about how research and health care decisions and regulations could be made, who could make them, and what their long-term implications would be. In the late 1960s, philosophers and theologians, physicians and lawyers, policymakers and legislators began to write about these questions, to hold conferences, to establish institutes, and to publish journals for the study of bioethics.

In 1969, the Institute of Society, Ethics, and the Life Sciences was established at Hastings-on-Hudson,

New York. Two years later, the Kennedy Institute of Ethics was established at Georgetown University, Washington DC. In 1973, the first edition of *The Hastings Center Studies* pointed out the problems and the needs:

> Remarkable advances are being made in organ transplantation, human experimentation, prenatal diagnosis of genetic disease, the prolongation of life and control of human behavior — and each advance has posed difficult problems requiring that scientific knowledge be matched by ethical insight.[3]

The federal government, private philanthropists and foundations, universities, medical schools, and committed professionals moved quickly to address these questions. The federal government supported programs through the National Science Foundation's EVIST (Ethics and Values in Science and Technology) and the National Endowment for the Humanities developed applied medical ethics courses for both medical students and college undergraduates. Both public and private universities established departments, institutes, or programs in bioethics, including some in which graduate studies could be pursued. Professional organizations (including local bar and medical associations) began to establish committees to look at ethical issues in health care. In addition, such interdisciplinary organizations as the Society for Health and Human Values came into existence, including among their members physicians, nurses, social workers, attorneys, theologians, and philosophers.

Hospitals, too, began to consider how bioethical concerns affected the care they provided patients. In 1976, the Massachusetts General Hospital Critical Care Committee published its recommendations for treating hopelessly ill patients and for using critical care facilities. In Roman Catholic hospitals, committees (often called medical-moral committees) were formed not only to discuss such specific care issues as sterilization, but also to consider the more general question of how Catholic values should be implemented in Catholic hospitals.

In November 1978, the President's Commission for the Study of Ethical Problems in Medicine and Medical and Biobehavioral Research was created; its members began work in January 1980. The United States Congress charged them to conduct studies and report on a number of topics, including the definition of death, informed consent, and access to health care. By spring 1984, the commission had published nine reports addressing many of the problems then facing the health care system. Building upon the work that had been done in the 1960s and 1970s, the commission looked to find where consensus existed and where serious disagreements and uncertainties still remained.

Their reports stand as a new foundation for the organized and socially sanctioned study of the ethical implications of high-technology medical care and of ethical regulation of the health care industry itself. The remainder of the 1980s may see reduced emphasis on protecting individual privacy and liberty rights, and increased emphasis on allocating resources and demonstrating the effectiveness of complex treatments, especially in terms of the quality of life that is achieved by prolonging life. The commission's work will make that transition in emphases more understandable.

The President's Commission, like the National Commission for the Protection of Human Subjects before it, established a model for finding consensus where it existed and for articulating ethical conflicts when consensus could not be found. They did for the nation what each ethics committee can do for its own hospital. Both commissions seriously studied the problems they addressed, listened attentively to those specialists who helped them to think about the issues, and withdrew in order to consider the questions from their own viewpoints. On most topics, they were then able to reach a consensus that enabled them to make recommendations that are both respected and influential. The process by which they achieved their final product is often discernible in the pages of the reports themselves. Their uncertainties and their disagreements are written in those documents. So also are their agreements and their reasoning.

Ethics committees are the next step in the unfolding of the bioethics movement. They will find answers no more easily than did earlier workers in these fields. The questions are, perhaps, growing even more difficult. Nevertheless, the work of ethics committees is made richer by those who wrote and thought about these matters in the past two decades. One of the first tasks of ethics committee members is to educate themselves. The existing body of work will provide the means for that task.

Development of Ethics Committees

In 1960, Belding Scribner, M.D., University of Washington, Seattle, introduced the shunt to medicine. The device made it possible to treat end-stage renal disease by long-term hemodialysis and, along the way, brought into being the first ethics committees. Because there were insufficient numbers of dialysis machines available between 1960 and 1972, all chronic kidney disease patients could not receive treatment.

Some patients were rejected because they did not meet medical criteria: they were too young or too old or they had other medical problems that made success with dialysis less likely. Others were out of luck because they did not live in states where dialysis was available. Scribner's treatment program, for example, admitted only Washington residents. But even with these restrictions, there were still more patients than dialysis machines.

In Seattle, Scribner's hospital formed a treatment committee whose membership included physicians, members of the hospital staff, and lay members of the community. The treatment committee's job was to review the cases of patients who were medically qualified for dialysis and to select from among them the one or two people who would actually receive treatment. Those who were not selected died. In 1962, *Life* magazine published a story about this anonymous committee and their selection processes. It was obvious that individuals were being selected for treatment (and thus for life) on the basis of criteria related to social worth, and charges of ethical insensitivity were leveled against the Seattle program. Scribner was astounded by the criticism because the committee had been established in response to the hospital's ethical concerns about selection. Treatment was not available for all who needed it; some selection method was necessary. What was wrong with a group of well-informed and responsible hospital and community members making sensitive, thoughtful choices?

By 1972, when the federal government chose to fund all treatment for end-stage renal disease, talk about treatment committees ceased. It is possible that some hospitals maintained or created treatment committees after 1972, using them to consider ethical problems in clinical care, but, if so, these committees have left no published records of their activities. In 1976, 14 years after *Life* had informed the world about ethics committees, the New Jersey Supreme Court's decision, *In the Matter of Karen Ann Quinlan,* reintroduced the topic. The New Jersey justices had been highly impressed by an article written by Karen Teel, M.D.[4] Teel's article discussed the value of hospital ethics committees for resolving clinical care dilemmas that had an ethical dimension. Teel asserted that "[many] hospitals have established an ethics committee . . . which serves to review the individual circumstances of ethical dilemmas and . . . [whose] status is more that of an advisory than of an enforcing body." It is unlikely that *many* hospitals had such committees, unless Teel is including the physician committees (used to approve abortions) as well as dialysis committees. Abortion committees were analogous to dialysis treatment committees insofar as patient

selection was the issue, but the dialysis treatment committees were multidisciplinary groups making self-acknowledged ethical, rather than medical, decisions. The abortion committees, on the other hand, had only doctors as members and were, at least on the face of it, making *medical* judgments about whether or not a patient's medical condition fit the state definition under which abortion could be performed legally. In any case, both abortion and dialysis committees had disappeared by 1976.

The justices, wrestling with the problem of whether or not Quinlan's respirator could be disconnected, found great merit in Teel's ethics committees, even though they did not appear to understand what such committees did or were supposed to do. In their landmark decision, they ruled that if Quinlan's attending physician determined that there was no reasonable chance that she would ever return to a "cognitive, sapient state," and *if a hospital ethics committee agreed with that prognosis,* then the life support apparatus could be withdrawn at her guardian's or family's request.

The ethics committees recommended by the *Quinlan* decision were not really ethics committees but were instead *prognosis* committees, dealing with medical descriptions and definitions, not moral ones. (The courts regularly compress medical and moral decisions into a single issue, thus making ethical matters even more difficult than they are on their own terms, and the *Quinlan* decision was not unusual in this respect.) Nevertheless, despite the decision's inherent confusion, it was widely publicized and many hospitals subsequently formed ethics committees, especially in New Jersey, where the *Quinlan* decision had legal force.

After *Quinlan,* the talk about ethics committees again subsided. In many hospitals, however, some doctors, nurses, hospital administrators, and social workers continued to worry about the increasing problems inherent in high-technology care. Some small groups began to form, usually calling themselves bioethics study groups. They met regularly to discuss the clinical problems they were facing, attended conferences on ethical problems in health care, and tried to interest their colleagues in addressing the problems in a systematic manner. Over time, as the groups educated themselves, some took on a more formal role in the hospital. They began to provide institutionwide education programs, to work on guidelines that would help to make decision making less traumatic, and, in a few hospitals, to offer their meetings as a forum in which individual health care professionals could discuss specific cases and specific treatment decisions. These groups worked unknown, for the most part, to one another or to the world.

Then, in 1982, the case of Baby Doe caused many to look again at ethics committees. In April of that year, a Down's syndrome infant with an esophageal atresia was born in Monroe County, Indiana. Some physicians involved in the infant's care recommended immediate surgical repair of the atresia, while others thought that treatment should not be offered because the infant's quality of life would not be good. They believed the baby should be allowed to die. The parents chose nontreatment. The baby died, but not before a series of court hearings, rulings, and appeals. As the infant died of starvation, Indiana judges at all levels affirmed the parents' right to choose nontreatment (as long as it was recommended by a physician) for their child. The case received widespread and, for the most part, negative publicity.

In the spring of 1983, the President's Commission for the Study of Ethical Problems in Medicine and Biomedical and Biobehavioral Research issued its report, *Deciding to Forego Life-Sustaining Treatment.* The 550-page report included chapters on making treatment decisions for incompetent patients and for seriously ill newborns. Realizing that there were ongoing ethical problems in these decisions, the commissioners suggested that hospitals themselves should provide procedures to "promote effective decision making" for incompetent patients. Hospital ethics committees seemed to them a reasonable, if untried, means for promoting effective decision making through education, policy recommendations, and case review. They realized, however, that ethics committees might create as many problems as they solved.[5]

Then, in the fall of 1983, the case of Baby Jane Doe arose in New York. This case, which involved parents who chose to refuse surgery for their child with spina bifida and hydrocephaly (opting instead for "conservative" treatment, including the use of antibiotics), kept the problem of treatment decisions for handicapped newborns firmly before the public. It demonstrated that both parents and doctors risked extensive legal involvement when treatment decisions were made in these gray areas, especially if life-prolonging or aggressive treatment was being withheld.

It was clear that these decisions required increased sensitivity to the ethical dimensions, improved education of the parents and the health care team about the practical implications of disabilities, specific hospital policies to assist the decision makers, and recognition that parents and doctors—those who held the legal responsibility for making these very difficult decisions—needed as much help as they could get in making the decision. From this need grew the recommendation, put forward both by the U.S. Department of Health and Human Services (DHHS) in the Baby Doe regulations (January 1984) and independently by the American Academy of Pediatrics, that each hospital providing newborn care, especially those with neonatal intensive care units (NICUs), form an infant care review committee. The recommendations made by DHHS and the American Academy of Pediatrics added to the President's Commission statement that generally endorsed the *idea* of ethics committees.

Others also believed that ethics committees could help health care providers and patients find their way out of the maze created by modern, technological medicine. Some state legislatures passed resolutions approving of hospital ethics committees, as did some state hospital associations, state medical associations, and insurance companies. At the national level, the American Hospital Association and the Catholic Hospital Association quickly made formal recommendations about hospital ethics committees being an appropriate or potential means for ensuring good decision-making practices. Eventually, even the American Medical Association endorsed ethics committees, although that organization and the American College of Physicians were concerned about the prospect of the committees intruding upon the doctor-patient relationship.[6]

A 1981 survey of hospitals produced for the President's Commission found that less than 1 percent of American hospitals had ethics committees,[7] but that figure included only ethics committees that were involved in decision making. More recent figures (1985) suggest that statistic may now be as high as 50 percent. One survey found that, among hospitals with NICUs, over half had committees by early 1985 and most of the others were considering forming them.[8] Little was known about those committees that did exist prior to 1984, when the rate of increase became so rapid. It was apparent that if many hospitals were to form such committees (and that committees were being rapidly formed was evident from the sudden appearance across the nation of well-attended conferences on ethics committees), they would pretty much have to pull themselves up by their own bootstraps. That in itself could be a problem but, if ethics committees did not yet know what they needed to know, they were not bogged down in a lot of old methods either. They had the virtue of being untried.

The President's Commission gave prominence to the idea of ethics committees at a fortuitous time. Although the bioethics community had been worrying about decisions to forego treatment for handicapped infants and terminally ill patients for many years, there had not been sufficient concern either within the health care industry or from the body politic to turn that concern into action. With the two Baby

Doe cases (as well as a number of movies, television programs, and other popular treatments of these issues), the question jelled and many more ethics committees were formed.

Although multidisciplinary groups in health care are a relatively new idea, ethics committees have some similarities to institutional review boards. An important difference, of course, is that IRBs are legally mandated and are empowered to make formal decisions. The IRBs appeared to have resolved the problems of ethically questionable research (although, as the President's Commission pointed out, there was distressingly little documentation on how IRBs functioned and on whether or not they were effective, and although they were certainly *perceived* to be "a good thing," that is, they didn't seem to stop the research process). Ethics committees appeared to be a good approach because they were sufficiently similar to other ways of solving problems involving conflicting moral values and because they had the potential for providing public involvement. Ethics committees could be a symbolic reminder that treatment decisions need to be consistent with overall social values. Furthermore, the committees could help doctors, nurses, patients, and families think about the nature of social values. Of course, the precise problem in many of these cases is that there is no consensus about which course of action is correct or which social values are most important. Thus, the "ethics committee model" is not a way of providing treatment decisions but rather a forum through which different values, perceptions, and information about treatment decisions can be discussed, assessed, and resolved by patients, their families, and the health care team. (See appendix A for example of ethics committee guidelines.)

Ethics committees now stand at a crucial point. They exist; they are being given institutional support and governmental encouragement. What they are to do and how they are to do it, however, has not been made very clear. Education, policy recommendation, and case review are their potential functions. For each, they will need to develop or refine specific skills. They will also need to define their own tasks carefully and to use their limited time and energy wisely. They must be able to bend their differences to find consensus, and yet preserve those differences so that they do not become rubber stamps for a single point of view. If they are effective, hospital ethics committees can be an important step in raising everyone's consciousness about the values by which we live and die.

Notes

1. The IRB is, in many respects, a direct ancestor of the ethics committee, insofar as it requires formation of a committee with both professional and lay representation to address ethical problems of medical activities. There are many differences between them, however. For example, IRBs have full veto power over all research because without their approval, public funding as well as, in many instances, private funding is unavailable. IRBs have clearly stated responsibilities and are mandated by federal action. In addition, IRBs are administrative review committees that customarily review written research protocols and informed consent documents. They rarely exercise their power to review ongoing research, whereas ethics committees often conduct case review.

2. A definition of irreversible coma. *JAMA*. 1968. 205:337.

3. *Hastings Cent Rep* 1973. 1(1):3.

4. Teel, Karen. The physician's dilemma. A doctor's view: What the law should be. *Baylor Law Rev* 1975. 27:6.

5. President's Commission for the Study of Ethical Problems in Medicine and Biomedical and Behavioral Research. *Deciding to Forego Life-Sustaining Treatment.* Washington, DC: U.S. Government Printing Office, 1983, pp. 160-9. Of the 11 reports of the commission, 4 are of primary interest to ethics committees and are discussed in a later chapter.

6. American College of Physicians. Ethics manual. *Ann Intern Med.* 1984. 101:129-37,263-74.

7. Younger, Stuart. A National Survey of Hospital Ethics Committees: Appendix F. *Critical Care Medicine.* 1983. 11(11):902-5.

8. Ethics committees double since 83: Survey, *Hospitals.* 1985. 59(21):60-64.

References

Glantz, L. Contrasting institutional review boards with institutional ethics committees. In: Cranford, R. E., and Doudera, A. E., eds. *Institutional Ethics Committees and Health Care Decision Making.* Ann Arbor, MI: Health Administration Press, 1984, pp. 129-37.

Hospital ethics committees surveyed. *Hospitals.* May 16, 1984. 58(8):50.

Jonsen, A., and Jameton, A. Bioethics, history. In: Reich, W. T., ed. *Encyclopedia of Bioethics,* New York: Free Press, 1978, pp. 992-1004.

Kalchbrenner, J., Kelly, M. J., and McCarthy, D. G. Ethics committees and ethicists in Catholic hospitals, *Hosp. Progr.* 1983. 64(9):47-51.

Rosner, F. Hospital medical ethics committees: a review of their development. *JAMA.* 1985. 253(18):2693-7.

Winslade, W. J., and Ross, J. W. *Choosing Life or Death.* New York: Free Press, 1986, pp. 23-51.

Youngner, S. J., Jackson, D. L., and others. A national survey of hospital ethics committees. *Critical Care Medicine.* 1983. 11(11):902-5.

Chapter 2

Ethical Context for Health Care

A concern with ethics implies a belief that one should lead a good life and that leading the good life means doing what is right. The obvious problem, of course, is knowing what is *right*. The prior problem is knowing what is *good*. Throughout the centuries, philosophers have been unable to agree about the correct way to identify and characterize what is good; we are no better off today in the search for the undisputed "truth" about *good* or about *right* and *wrong* conduct. Nevertheless, the lack of general agreement about what good defines the good life, or about how to identify right and wrong actions, does not mean that any feeling or opinion about what is right is as acceptable or good as any other. Because ethics involves analytic approaches, any statement about ethical decision making in a particular instance implies reasons, explanations, and goals that can be clearly articulated. A conclusion is justified by the clarity and consistency of the relationship between reasons, value assumptions, and goals. It is not sufficient to say, "Well, that is my opinion and we are all entitled to our own opinions."

All ethical systems do not agree upon a single good that is being sought. In fact, not only do the systems differ from each other in their ideas about what constitutes the good, but many systems have more than one primary value, and thus may not be internally consistent. They may believe that the object of the good life is pleasure, happiness, freedom, knowledge, love, or some combination of these or other values. Many disagreements about moral judgments arise when two people who have different goals (or primary values) try to decide which act is the right act. For example, a researcher may hold the acquisition of knowledge (or truth) as a primary goal, whereas an animal-rights activist may believe that the pursuit of knowledge does not justify causing pain to animals. They may have difficulty resolving their differences about whether a specific research protocol is ethical, because one aims at avoiding unjustified pain and the other aims at acquiring potentially useful information.

Cultures, religions, institutions, professions, and individuals may each have a unique idea about what constitutes the good that is to be pursued by right action. To make matters more confusing, an individual can and is likely to accept the goals of more than one system, which may lead to significant problems of conflicting values.

Ethical analysis falls broadly into two branches: deontological systems and teleological systems. Different systems may share the same values (that is, definitions of good) or they may have different values. *Deontological systems* are those in which the rightness of the act depends upon the act itself. Thus, for example, a system might hold (as most religious systems do) that taking a human life (or an innocent human life) is wrong. It is not wrong because it hurts people, or because it is unaesthetic, or because it makes the living unhappy, although all of those may be true statements. It is wrong either because God has forbidden it or, for nontheistically based ethical systems, because it is inherently wrong, intuitively wrong, or a violation of natural law. That is, killing an innocent person is wrong in *principle*. Deontological systems depend upon principles and, often, upon rules. (Principles are statements of general truths; rules, on the other hand, are specific obligations.) The Ten Commandments of *The Bible* are good examples of straightforward deontological rules. Exceptions are not granted.

Teleological systems, unlike deontological systems, are focused on the *consequences* of acts. Such systems are often referred to as *consequentialist ethics.* Here, the rightness of an act depends upon what happens as a result of the act. Thus, teleologists may believe that, in general, killing is wrong; in order to assess its rightness or wrongness correctly, however, one would have to look at the consequences of the specific killing or the class of killings. Whether the killing was wrong would depend upon the consequences of the act. Thus, to kill one to save many might be permissible, even if that one were innocent. Terrorists with hostages could use this kind of justification, even though they might consistently believe that killing, in general, is wrong. Similarly, those who believe in mercy killing could justify the act in terms of its consequences: that it ended suffering or that, in some cases, it served human freedom.

Both the researcher and the animal-rights activist in the earlier example were deontologists who disagreed about the primary good. A conflict between a deontologist and a consequentialist can be demonstrated by their disagreement about truth-telling. The deontologist may believe that one should always tell the truth, even though that path may sometimes lead to unhappiness, anger, or other negative results. The consequentialist, on the other hand, measures the results of the truth-telling and thereby determines whether it is morally appropriate to tell the truth in any given situation.

Consequentialists can be divided into subgroups. The two groups that are most familiar today are *ethical egoists* and *utilitarians. Ethical egoism* states that one has an obligation to do whatever will produce good for oneself. The good is unspecified and may appear to others as either noble or ignoble. For example, it might be defined as achieving money, power, or personal popularity or it might be defined as achieving union with God. Ethical egoism is very common today in America and is compatible with the contemporary American emphasis on individualism.

Utilitarianism is the philosophy based upon the writings of Jeremy Bentham and John Stuart Mill. Utilitarian thinking is very common and is frequently the ethical basis of institutional policies. Many variations of utilitarianism exist, but, in general, each asserts that the good is pleasure (but considers pleasure to be of a higher kind than mere sensual pleasures) and that right actions are those that provide the greatest good (sometimes the greatest net good) for the greatest number. Utilitarians are obliged to be balancers: they must calculate the pleasure produced by an act against the misery it produces and decide where the balance lies. Utilitarianism implies some ability to quantify pleasures and miseries but it is often unclear about how those who espouse this view are to make such evaluations. Generally, utilitarians also base their calculations beyond the moment; that is, they consider the long-term benefits and burdens as well as the immediate ones. Most utilitarians appear to base their calculus on intuitive rather than quantitative judgments about how much pleasure and pain are involved in various choices. It is difficult to *count* pleasure and pain in order to demonstrate that one exceeds the other, although economists who work on utilitarian principles have tried to measure pleasures and pains more concretely, albeit indirectly.

In both deontological (principled) and teleological (consequentialist) systems, ethical dilemmas can arise when values, principles, or rules conflict with reference to a single action. In health care, ethical dilemmas can arise either because there is a conflict of values within an individual decision maker's ethical system, or because there are multiple decision makers and their various ethical systems are in conflict (or a combination of both). If a physician believes that the goals of medicine are to preserve life and to prevent pain and suffering, there will be an ethical dilemma if an action preserves one value but violates the other. For example, continuing to provide food and fluids for a conscious but acutely senile and bedridden patient may preserve life, but it may inflict further pain and suffering as a result of pressure sores and general misery from living such a constricted life. For some health care workers dealing with such a case, preserving life is the primary value and preventing pain and suffering is a secondary value; thus, an apparent conflict can be easily resolved because the primary value rules. (Many assumptions are involved in this statement. The dilemma would be easily resolved if the person were a deontologist, or if he or she were a consequentialist and the amount of pain from continuing to live did not greatly exceed the good of continued life, a good that might be largely symbolic, but no less a good.) An example of ethical systems in conflict is presented when a physician believes that his or her primary duty is to keep the patient alive (to preserve life), but the patient's primary value is freedom or autonomy to act as he or she wishes, even if life is thereby shortened. Ethical conflicts and dilemmas can involve not only what decision should be made but also who should make that decision.

The primary values that are used in making moral decisions in health care are patient autonomy, health care provider beneficence (doing good), health care provider nonmaleficence (doing no harm), and justice (or fairness—generally, treating similar cases similarly). These values or principles are discussed more fully later in this chapter under "Ethical Principles in Health Care." In the United States, enormous emphasis is placed on individual autonomy as a primary value. Thus, the wishes of competent patients can rarely be overridden, and only then with very powerful justifications. It is because we place such emphasis on the value of autonomous choice that decisions about incompetent patients (who have not made their wishes about treatment known when they were competent) are so difficult for us. We are frequently at a loss as to how to evaluate the relative importance of secondary values when the primary value of patient autonomy does not apply.

Psychological Views of Moral Development

In recent years, psychologists have looked at many of the same questions that philosophers have perennially pondered, but from their own professional perspective. Their theories of moral development permit us to learn something else about how moral disagreements develop, how to untangle them, and even how to learn from the disagreements. Lawrence Kohlberg, a professor at Harvard University, is the preeminent moral-development theorist, but his thinking grew out of Jean Piaget's writings on children's intellectual development. His theories are descriptive, rather than proven facts. Others in this field have taken issue with his categories, arguing that they are based too exclusively on rights-oriented ethics and do not take into account other ethical approaches, particularly those based on responsibility for others.[1]

Kohlberg postulates that there are six (or perhaps seven) stages of moral development and that humans go through them in much the same way that infants learn first to roll over, then to sit up, then to crawl, and finally to walk. There are two important correlates of Kohlberg's system: first, everyone goes through the stages in the same order, but not everyone goes through all the stages; second, a person at one stage can understand the reasoning of any stage below him or her, but can understand no more than one stage above. These correlates, especially the latter one, are important when it comes to assessing the nature of disagreements about ethical judgments.[2]

Kohlberg has characterized these stages in a number of ways, but perhaps the easiest way to remember them is by the differing kinds of justifications employed in the various stages:

- When a person making a stage 1 decision is asked why that is the right decision, he or she would reply, "Because if I do not make that decision I will be punished."
- When a person making a stage 2 decision is asked why that is the right decision, he or she would reply, "Because if I make that decision, I will be rewarded and other people will help me." This is perhaps best characterized by a "you scratch my back and I'll scratch yours" philosophy.
- A stage 3 decision maker replies, "Others whom I care about will be pleased if I do this because they have taught me that this is what a good person does."
- At Stage 4, the decision maker offers explanations that demonstrate his or her role in society and how decisions further the social order (for example, obeying the law makes life more orderly).
- At Stage 5, the decision maker justifies decisions by explaining that acts will contribute to social well-being and that each member of society has an obligation to every other member.
- Stage 6 decisions are justified by appeals to personal conscience and universal ethical principles.

It is important to understand that Kohlberg's system does not help us to find "right" answers, as do ethical theories. Instead, it shows us how people get to their answers. As a result, if you asked the same question of someone at each of the six levels, the answer might be the same in all cases, but the explanation for the decision would be different. As an example, suppose a terminally ill man in great pain asked a doctor or nurse for enough barbiturates to commit suicide.

- The stage 1 health care provider might reply, "No, because I could lose my license if anybody found out I had done that."
- The stage 2 doctor or nurse might answer, "No, because if I became known as a doctor or nurse who did that kind of thing, other doctors and nurses might not refer patients to me."
- The stage 3 doctor or nurse could reply, "No, because that's against the law and professionals should obey the law," or "No, because my colleagues would no longer respect me if they knew I had done that."
- At stage 4, the reply could be, "No, because if everyone did that, then doctors and nurses would no longer be trusted to save lives."
- At stage 5, "No, even though the patient might suffer less, we need to be faithful to our respect for life because otherwise we might lose our standards and abuse our authority."

- Finally, a stage 6 decision might be explained as "No, because I personally believe that no one has a right to take his or her own life and thus I cannot be party to such an action."

Note again that the stages do not determine the decision. A set of yes answers could also be written for each of these stages. For example, stage 1 reasoning might argue that if the patient continues to live, he is only going to make life miserable for all the staff; on the other hand, a stage 2 decision to provide help with the suicide might be justified by the comment that because the patient was paying for technical advice, the doctor or nurse ought to provide help to him or her, as long as the patient was not asking the doctor or nurse to cause his or her death directly. A stage 5 thinker might argue that no one benefits from keeping individuals alive longer than they want to live, and a stage 6 answer might be that the decision to exit life is such a serious one that it needs to be honored if it is made reasonably.

These categories can give ethics committee members a second way of seeing how ethical discussions sometimes get bogged down. A person who is capable of stage 4 reasoning, for example, may be reasoning at any level below that, but he or she will be nonplussed by someone who is trying to use a stage 6 argument. Ideally, if discussion is to be effective or bring about consensus or agreement, the discussants should be talking on the same level of ethical discourse. In many ethics committees, there is a belief that once the state of the law has been established, the ethical problem has been answered. That is, however, typical stage 4 (and sometimes stage 3) thinking; members would do well to address the question on a more complex ethical level. Furthermore, the belief that the law speaks clearly and unambiguously is often a mistaken one because the law, too, embodies various stages of ethical development. The U.S. Supreme Court, for example, when addressing questions of constitutional law, usually demonstrates aspects of stage 4 and stage 6 decision making, but other decisions can be seen as stage 3 or stage 4.

Whenever a committee addresses a particular policy or case, the members need to be sure that they are clear about what values they hold, both individually and as a group, and where the conflict lies. Is it between the values, principles, or rules that lie within a single ethical system? Is it between values, principles, or rules that belong to different ethical systems? When consensus has been reached, the members should be aware of the stage level of the decision. An ethics committee ought not to be using stages 2 and 3 reasoning for cases or issues as critical as those that

usually come before the committee. Stage 5, which includes a concern for everyone's welfare and the protection of everyone's rights, does not seem too high a level for which to aim. It is unlikely that everyone will accept the final decision for the same reasons, but members should be aware of the level of their own reasons and, to the extent that it is possible, of the level of others.

Ethical Principles in Health Care

Ethical principles in health care stem from the assumption that there must be respect for persons. There are then three derived principles (or four, depending upon how they are conceptualized) that ethics committee members should be concerned with in their work: *autonomy, beneficence* and/or *nonmaleficence,* and *justice.* When these principles come into conflict, decision making must be careful, reflective, and well-articulated.

We respect *autonomy* when we refrain from interfering with peoples' opportunities to control their own lives by making their own choices. Autonomy refers to personal choice, control, and self-definition. Autonomy assumes the existence of individual values that do not need to be shared by others in order to be worthy of respect. In health care, patient autonomy is seen as the patient's right to receive accurate information about his or her health and treatment; to be fully informed not only about the physician's recommendations but also about alternative treatments that might preserve life, prevent disease, and relieve suffering; and to choose or to refuse any of those treatments. In addition, patient autonomy is served by permitting patients to choose others to hold and receive information and to make their decisions for them, whether physician, family member, or attorney-in-fact (as in the circumstance of granting durable power of attorney).

According to some writers, the principle of *beneficence* (doing good) is separate from the principle of *nonmaleficence* (causing no harm).[3] In this conception, doing good is a principle of equal importance to that of not causing harm. Others believe that beneficence is a fundamental principle that includes nonmaleficence as an aspect of the principle.[4] When beneficence is seen as the inclusive principle, it may be regarded as having four aspects: (1) one should not do evil or should not cause harm to another; (2) one should prevent evil or harm to another; (3) one should remove evil or sources of harm to another; and (4) one should promote good. These aspects can be ranked in importance and conflicts are then resolved by that ranking. According to Frankena, the listing given above is the rank order of importance. Thus, if one must choose between not causing harm or doing good, then one should choose not to cause harm. Similarly, preventing harm is preferable to removing harm.

The final principle is that of *justice*. Justice has many aspects but in health care the aspect of concern is usually distributive justice, that is, how burdens and benefits should be distributed. Even though a child is brought up to be concerned with fairness, he or she will often find it very difficult to decide what constitutes fairness. Fairness and justice are not interchangeable terms in all contexts, although they are often used that way. A choice might seem unfair to an individual but, in terms of social values, would be just. For example, affirmative action might be seen as just with respect to society, even though it is unfair to some individuals. When there are insufficient resources (whether they be vaccine serum, nursing care, or donated hearts), distributive justice is concerned with how the resources are to be allocated among those who are in need. Should all receive the same amount, even if no one receives enough? Should those who can best profit from sufficient resources (for example, those who are most likely to be returned to socially productive lives) receive all they need, while others receive little or none? Should sufficient resources be available to all who can pay for them? Should adequate resources be provided first for those who are least able to help themselves? All these are questions of distributive justice. There is no necessary reason why, for example, "the greatest good for the greatest number" should prevail when issues of justice are considered. As Beauchamp and Childress point out, "justice" means that we should treat every person fairly and that everyone should receive what he or she needs or deserves (although that is not always possible). These terms all need to be defined, however, in the context of any single decision involving claims of justice.

In general, patient autonomy is considered to be the most important of the three principles in health care decision making at the patient care level. Justice or beneficence, however, may receive higher priority at governmental policy levels. The constitutional right of privacy and the informed consent doctrine are both based upon the principle of autonomy. Patient autonomy means that the preferences of competent patients are to be accepted as long as they understand the implications of their choices and the alternative choices that are open to them. This is not an absolute value, for there are times when respecting a patient's autonomy may cause great hardship to others, giving rise to

questions of justice or beneficence. For example, there have been instances in which the parents of young children have refused, for religious reasons, to consent to blood transfusions that they themselves needed. Courts have sometimes overruled patient preferences in such cases because harm would come to the minor children if their parent was allowed to die (nonmaleficence) or because the state's duty was to protect the minor children (beneficence). The state, as protector of the minor children, can make this decision. Similarly, as protector of all citizens, the state might choose to overrule patient preferences in such cases to protect society in general from having to take on responsibility for the care of these parents' children (justice).

Involuntary treatment of mental patients is another circumstance in which beneficence may outweigh autonomy considerations. Mental illness itself is not a priori evidence of incompetency but patients who are involuntarily committed are routinely treated without their consent and even against their wishes. Similarly, public health measures may involve individuals undergoing tests and treatment they do not voluntarily choose, for the protection of others as well as themselves.

Beneficence and nonmaleficence frequently come into conflict when medical care can either extend life or cause suffering, or both. Thus, a patient with advanced, terminal cancer may be offered further chemotherapy that can prolong life but will also involve additional pain and suffering. Generally, patient autonomy is used to resolve conflicts between doing good and causing harm. Sometimes, however, autonomy cannot be exercised (as in cases of incompetent patients, especially when they have never been competent). If the principle of autonomy cannot be used to resolve the conflict, then the two are frequently "balanced" and the relationship between the amount of good done and the amount of harm done is roughly estimated.

Both justice and beneficence might also be of greater weight than patient autonomy in "temporary" decisions. That is, suppose a patient with a serious, chronic illness is informed that yet another complication has arisen. For example, a long-term dialysis patient is advised that amputation of a gangrenous limb is necessary. First, the patient refuses to consent to the operation because he cannot accept yet another restriction on his life; then he refuses to consent to further dialysis. The patient may be fully competent in the ordinary sense of the word: he understands the nature of his condition and the need for both the dialysis and the amputation, as well as the implications of refusing one or both. Giving primacy to patient autonomy would suggest that the refusal should be respected — it is an informed refusal from a competent patient. Yet beneficence would suggest that this refusal should not be accepted too quickly.

A patient receiving such hard news almost inevitably undergoes severe stress and may react only on the basis of his or her feelings. It may be that ultimately the patient's autonomy will be respected and the refusal will be honored. Yet, health care professionals' obligations of beneficence are such that they should pursue some kind of temporizing measures in order to ensure that refusing treatment is the patient's genuine desire. In general, whenever respecting patient autonomy leads to the patient's death or to serious harm, the principle of beneficence obligates those involved to be very sure not only that the patient is competent but that the patient's wishes come from thoughtful reflection, not through emotional crisis. Jay Katz, a psychiatrist at Yale School of Law, suggests that a physician ought never to accept (on the basis of patient autonomy) a patient's refusal of either curative or ameliorative treatment unless the patient is able to articulate the reasons for refusal and unless the physician is able to understand those reasons, even if he or she does not agree with the patient.[5] This would be even more important if the patient were incompetent and a family member was refusing curative or ameliorative treatment on the patient's behalf.

Language of Bioethics

Bioethics, like any other area of study, has its own vocabulary, although its language is perhaps more eclectic than that of other fields. Because it has developed in an interdisciplinary setting, it tends to have gathered up language from medicine, philosophy, theology, law, and ordinary life. Individuals working in this area need to be particularly careful to make sure they understand the meaning of frequently used terms because ordinary language is often used to convey technical information. Furthermore, because life and death and strongly held values are frequently at issue, the language bears a heavy emotional burden. When discussing ethical problems of health care, committee members should use language precisely and should be sure they understand one another's meanings. Such terms as *brain death, permanent unconsciousness, persistent vegetative state, cortical death, neocortical death, irreversible coma,* and *whole brain death* are often used as if they were all more or less interchangeable words, though they are not. Similarly, *living will, natural death act directive,* and *durable power of attorney* are used as if they all referred to the same phenomenon. They do not. Language sometimes reveals conceptual problems in this area (the contradiction involved in *living will*), but sometimes it may as easily obscure those problems (comments that *a brain dead person has died*).

Previous sections explained the use of such terms as deontology, teleology/consequentialism, autonomy, beneficence, and so forth. This section includes others, many of which have common meanings. The importance of most of these terms lies in how they are used in relation to other terms used in bioethics.

Euthanasia, Suicide, and Assisted Suicide

Euthanasia comes from the Greek and means, literally, *good death.* Technically, it refers to a death under two conditions: first, it comes earlier than is necessary, given the capabilities of medicine, and, second, it is intended by those parties who either act to hasten the death or fail to act to postpone it (health care professionals, patients and/or family members). Commonly, however, euthanasia is most frequently used to refer to "mercy killing" or "active euthanasia." Active euthanasia means an action taken by someone other than the patient with the intention of ending the patient's life. Mercy killing or active euthanasia is usually considered murder. "Passive euthanasia" means allowing someone to die when there are means to prolong life and is not usually considered murder.

Euthanasia is distinguished from both suicide and assisted suicide. In euthanasia, a person other than the patient commits the act that leads to the patient's death. In suicide, it is the patient who commits the act that leads directly to death. In assisted suicide, a person other than the patient provides the patient with the means of death, but it is the patient who actually performs the act. Thus, if a physician intentionally gives a dying patient a fatal dose of medicine, it is euthanasia. If the dying patient gathers up a supply of sleeping pills and dies by taking these pills, it is suicide. If the health care professional provides the patient with a supply of drugs, knowing that the patient will probably use them to end his or her life, it is assisted suicide.

It is difficult to say much about euthanasia and obtain agreement. There is widespread fear and disapproval of euthanasia in American society and, depending upon definitions, the emotional levels of discussion about euthanasia may be significantly heightened. Beyond the distinctions mentioned, agreement becomes difficult. It is our advice that the term not be used and that discussions about the meaning of and differences between active, passive, voluntary, nonvoluntary, and involuntary euthanasia be redirected. Whatever the problem is, it is more effectively discussed in some vocabulary other than that of euthanasia.

Withholding Treatment and Withdrawing Treatment

The report of the President's Commission on this general topic used the phrase *foregoing treatment* to refer to both withholding and withdrawing treatment. Many health care professionals insist there is a significant difference between withholding treatment initially and withdrawing it after it has been initiated.[6]

Philosophers believe that there are no moral distinctions to be drawn between the permissibility of withholding and withdrawing. There may be psychological differences and legal differences, but these do not translate into moral differences. It is unethical to forego treatment that would be beneficial, but one is never obliged to provide treatment that is not beneficial. (This assumes that there are no other factors involved, such as the patient's wishes, promises to the patient, policies with respect to scarce resources, and so forth.) Frequently, of course, treatment is initiated because it is not certain whether it will be beneficial. Once that determination is made, however, the decision to continue or withdraw treatment should be based upon the patient's wishes and the benefit to the patient. Conflicts occur, of course, when little or no benefit can be expected but the patient or family members wish treatment to continue despite the absence of benefit. The opposite can occur as well, when the patient wishes treatment withdrawn even though the physicians believe that some benefit is available. These can be very difficult dilemmas, especially when resources are limited or benefits appear to be considerable.

Intended versus Unintended but Foreseeable Consequences

The question sometimes arises as to whether or not physicians should be able to administer a symptom-relieving drug, such as a pain killer, knowing that the drug may cause or accelerate the patient's death—even though the death is not an outcome sought by the physician or the patient. In this instance, the goal of prolonging life is in conflict with the goal of relieving suffering. Especially when a patient is terminally ill, the goal of relieving suffering ordinarily takes precedence. Therefore, the unintended consequence of death is justified when the intended consequence of relieving suffering is achieved. Clearly, the decision makers need to consider the full range of foreseeable effects and to weigh the risks of harm against the opportunity for benefit.

Suicide and Refusing Treatment

There are no hard-and-fast lines between suicide and refusing treatment. One difference that has been suggested focuses on analyzing the patient's intent. If the patient's primary purpose is to end his or her life, then the action can be construed as suicide. If, on the other hand, the intent is to avoid severe burdens, including pain and suffering, and death is the only way to achieve that end or is incidental to achieving that goal, then the action does not constitute suicide. Another distinction suggested by Professor Albert Jonsen, University of California, San Francisco School of Medicine, is that the patient who is refusing treatment is acknowledging that there is treatment available that will make it possible to continue living, but that he or she does not wish to take advantage of that assistance. Thus, treatment refusal includes both an acknowledgment of the existence of effective help and a refusal of that help. The suicide, on the other hand, takes the position that there is no help available and therefore there is no choice. Professor Jonsen has further suggested that when there is ambivalence about whether there is or is not help available to the individual, then that ambivalence probably indicates that the refusal is more likely a desire for suicide than for refusing treatment.[7]

Other health care providers, however, have suggested that almost all patients are ambivalent about refusing treatment. The distinction between suicide and refusing treatment is, alas, not an easy or clear one in some cases, especially when no terminal illness is involved. The case of Elizabeth Bouvia, for example, has some elements of both. Bouvia was a young adult, quadriplegic woman who asked that she be allowed to starve herself to death in the hospital while the hospital staff provided her with necessary supportive care, including pain medication. A court determined that the hospital and the physicians were not obliged to comply with her request and were, in fact, permitted to force feed her against her wishes in order to save her life.[8]

Deciding whether a patient's action constitutes a refusal of treatment or an embrace of suicide is especially problematic insofar as health care professionals are both legally and morally obligated to defer to patient preferences, on the one hand, but are legally and perhaps morally forbidden to assist a patient's suicide, on the other hand. As a practical matter, decisions to refuse life-saving treatment that appear suddenly or appear in response to some kind of crisis should not be immediately accepted at face value as autonomous refusal-of-treatment decisions. The implications of labeling a decision either a wish for suicide or an autonomous refusal of treatment are great, both for the patient and for the health care professionals, and the decision must be carefully considered.

Ordinary, Extraordinary, and Heroic Treatment; Proportionate and Disproportionate Treatment; and Beneficial and Nonbeneficial Treatment

Frequently it is said that a question about whether or not treatment should be provided can be answered on the basis of whether the treatment is ordinary or extraordinary (or heroic). The assumption is that ordinary treatment must always be used, whereas extraordinary or heroic treatment is optional. This terminology attempts to capture important moral distinctions but it is generally unsuccessful in doing so effectively. The President's Commission has provided an extensive discussion of these terms.[9] The commission concludes that the "ordinary-extraordinary" distinction should be rejected because the terms are neither defined nor used consistently. "Extraordinary," for example, is variously defined as nonstandard, unusual, invasive, risky, complex, expensive, or unlikely to be effective. None of these meanings alone facilitates a moral analysis of whether or not a particular treatment should be used.

In contrast, the "proportionate-disproportionate" distinction is amenable to more precise definitions and more consistent use, although it too may involve impressionistic assessments that are difficult to justify when there is disagreement. Furthermore, it is not always the case that proportionateness or disproportionateness is judged by an objective balancing of burdens and benefits. In the *Quinlan* case, for example, there may have been no burden to the patient from continued treatment, but treatment could nevertheless be withdrawn because there was little or, perhaps, no benefit to her. The assessment of burden and benefit must generally be made by the patient. Thus, a treatment that imposed a very great hardship on a patient, but also offered a considerable hope of benefit, would not be required if the patient believed the burden was greater than he or she wished to accept. A patient might, for example, refuse chemotherapy or dialysis as imposing too great a burden. Similarly, a treatment that offers little hope of benefit is not required even if it imposes no particular burden upon the patient. This area continues to exhibit difficulties and considerable ambiguity, primarily because its formulation depends upon the subjective interpretation of burden and benefit. There can be considerable differences of opinion among patients, families, and health care professionals as to how to estimate burdens and benefits.

Care and Treatment

Concerns about how to distinguish between ordinary care and medical treatment have risen recently with respect to artificial means of providing food and fluids, both to incompetent patients whose deaths are imminent and to incompetent patients for whom continued, but very "low-quality," life can be expected. (These cases range from terminal-stage cancer patients, to permanently unconscious patients, to seriously ill newborns, to severely senile patients who are bedridden.) Some courts have stated that physicians may regard artificial forms of feeding as they would any other form of medical treatment, at least in some situations. Although there is an undeniable logic to this position, many feel that logic is not sufficient to resolve the issue. Some persons assert that feeding is a basic human need, however it is achieved. Others argue that, because intravenous tubes, nasogastric tubes, and gastrostomy feeding are technological and invasive, they are not really comparable to hand feeding or to keeping the mouth and lips moistened. In trying to understand whether or not this distinction has any moral significance, one should also remember that providing food and fluids has significant psychological importance to those who care for these patients. Furthermore, it has symbolic importance to all current and future patients. For these reasons, its moral significance cannot be limited to a narrow logical analysis. For legal opinions, see the cases of *Barber v. Superior Court* and *In the Matter of Claire Conroy* in chapter 14.

Notes

1. See, especially, Gilligan, Carol. *In a Different Voice.* Cambridge, MA: Harvard University Press, 1982.

2. Boyce, W.D., and Jensen, L.C. *Moral Reasoning.* Lincoln: University of Nebraska Press, 1979, pp. 98-109.

3. Beauchamp T., and Childress, J. *Principles of Biomedical Ethics.* New York: Oxford University Press, 1979.

4. Frankena, W. K., *Ethics,* Englewood Cliffs, NJ: Prentice-Hall, 1973.

5. Katz, J. *The Silent World of Doctor and Patient.* 1984.

6. Law professor Nancy Rhoden has suggested that the major difference between the treatment of very low birthweight babies in this country and their treatment in England is that American physicians are much less willing to stop treatment once they have started than are their British counterparts (unpublished manuscript).

7. Comments made at the Conference on Emerging Issues in Bioethics, Los Angeles, November 9, 1984.

8. In 1986, the California appellate court held that Ms. Bouvia was entitled to refuse the nasogastric tube feedings recommended by her physician. Many disagree about whether this decision, which affirmed a competent patient's right to refuse treatment, means that a patient can commit suicide by refusing treatment. The California Supreme Court declined to review the case (*Bouvia v. Superior Court of Los Angeles,* No. B 019134, April 16, 1986).

9. President's Commission for the Study of Ethical Problems in Medicine and Biomedical and Behavioral Research, *Deciding to Forego Life-Sustaining Treatment,* Washington, DC: U.S. Government Printing Office, 1983, pp. 82-90.

References

Allen, D. F., and Fowler, M. D. Cognitive moral development theory and moral decisions for health care. *Law, Med Health Care.* 1982. 10(1):19-23.

Beauchamp, T., and Childress, J. *Principles of Biomedical Ethics,* 2nd ed. New York: Oxford University Press, 1983.

Veatch, R. M. From cases to rules: the challenge in contemporary medical ethics. In: Abernethy, V., ed. *Frontiers in Medical Ethics.* Cambridge, MA: Ballinger, 1980, pp. 43-62.

Chapter 3

The President's Commission and Its Reports

The President's Commission for the Study of Ethical Problems in Medicine and Biomedical and Behavioral Research began its work in 1980. It was intended to provide a temporary, national body that would consider the increasingly problematic situations that had arisen in medicine primarily, but not exclusively, as a result of advances in medical technology. The multidisciplinary, 10-person commission was chaired by attorney Morris Abrams, professor of law, New York University. Its staff director was Alexander Capron (currently Topping Professor of Law at the University of Southern California School of Law). During its three-year tenure, the commission held public hearings throughout the country, commissioned research studies and reports on a variety of topics, and published nine well-documented reports on the medical-legal-ethical issues that seemed most pressing. The commission functioned at a national level as a type of super-ethics committee. The reports are well-written, thorough, and thoughtful, and provide practical decision-making policies, principles, and guidelines. They can be of use both to health policy makers who are making decisions for society at large and to individual ethics committees and physicians who are deciding or making recommendations in individual cases. Already, court decisions routinely cite these reports as authoritative statements on bioethics issues.

Ethics committee members would do well to familiarize themselves with all the commission's reports, but they should be particularly familiar with four of them: *Defining Death (1981), Deciding to Forego Life-Sustaining Treatment (1983), Making Health Care Decisions, 3 vols. (1982-3),* and *Securing Access to Health Care, 3 vols. (1983).* These reports cover the topics that are most likely to be the primary focus for ethics committees during the next few years.

Deciding to Forego Life-Sustaining Treatment discusses treatment decisions for incompetent patients in general, for permanently unconscious patients in particular, and for seriously ill newborns, as well as decisions about cardiopulmonary resuscitation and do-not-resuscitate (DNR) orders. The report includes not only analyses of the problems but also specific recommendations and conclusions about who should make decisions to forego treatment and how those decisions should be made. The commission's recommendations do not have the force of law; they are only recommendations. To the extent that courts embrace them and legislatures act upon them, they will become law. However, they are very thoughtful and well-articulated judgments and ethics committees would be advised to be very concerned about having clear justifications for any recommendations, guidelines, or policies that are in opposition to either the letter or the spirit of the commission's recommendations.

As a result of the passage of 20 years and the excellent work of the President's Commission, consensus has been reached on some issues. However, even though both consensus and legislation exist on such topics as determination of death by brain-death criteria, clinical practices are not always consistent with either consensus or law. Thus, even in areas where what should be done is fairly clear, ethics committees need to persist in their educational efforts. In matters about which consensus has not been reached, education, policy-making, and consultation are made more difficult, but the need for them is just as great.

The following pages briefly summarize conclusions and recommendations from these President's Commission reports and then comment on the topic.

Brain-Death Criteria

In *Defining Death,* the President's Commission concludes that the restatement of the definition of death, including both brain-death criteria and heart-lung criteria, should be established by uniform state statute. The commission endorsed the Uniform Determination of Death Act. The report also includes a discussion of the arguments advanced as to redefining death with respect to "whole brain" and "higher brain" (neocortical) functioning.

Commentary. The redefinition of death was one of the earliest issues taken up in bioethics and there is general consensus about what is to be done, if not always about how to do it. Originally, the brain-death issue was closely tied to concerns about transplantation. Physicians feared that they risked murder charges if they removed organs before making a declaration of death; yet they risked ineffective transplants if they waited until heart-lung death occurred with the patient still connected to the respirator. Concerns about pronouncing death by brain-death criteria had a separate importance as well, however, because many believed that patients were being inappropriately kept on life-support systems when death by heart-lung criteria was inevitable within a fairly short period of time. This continued use of life-support was felt to be not only an inappropriate use of scarce resources but also an improper way to treat the patient or the body.

Over the past 15 years, the brain-death criteria for declaring death have been sharply refined, and the President's Commission includes the report of their medical consultants on appropriate brain-death criteria (*Defining Death,* 1981, appendix F). These standards are considerably more refined than those put forward in 1968 by the Harvard Medical School ad hoc committee. States with brain-death criteria statutes usually refer to the appropriate criteria as those "determined by accepted medical standards."

The primary medical considerations involving brain-death criteria include establishing standards for diagnosis and ensuring the certainty of the diagnosis. Hospitals should have policies establishing the appropriate criteria for the determination of brain death. This is, however, a matter of medical judgment. Ethical considerations with respect to brain-death criteria arise around the question of stopping treatment once brain-death criteria are met and death is declared. Many physicians continue to treat patients who meet brain-death criteria if the families do not consent to stopping treatment. Because the body has the appearance of life, some may believe that "treatment" should be continued. The commission concludes that there is no ethical reason to act differently toward these dead patients merely because their death is manifested in a different form. Dead bodies ought not to receive treatment because doing so suggests that they are still alive. Ethics committees may want to consider developing policies about stopping treatment for those who are declared dead by brain-death criteria. These will be useful in those instances in which the family objects to stopping treatment even though a patient meets brain-death criteria. Given the existence of brain-death statutes and the consensus about the appropriateness of these criteria as a basis for declaring death, there is no need to ask permission of the family to stop treatment. This does not, of course, preclude dealing compassionately with the family's needs to adjust to the reality of the patient's death.

Foregoing Treatment

Competent Patients

In *Deciding to Forego Life-Sustaining Treatment,* the President's Commission concludes that health care professionals have an obligation to "enhance patients' abilities to make decisions on their own behalf and to promote understanding of the available treatment options" (p. 3). They also conclude that there should be a presumption in favor of sustaining life: any decision that goes against this presumption should be carefully evaluated. In addition, they point out that although patient autonomy is a fundamental value, it is not an absolute one. The commission restricts patient autonomy in the following ways. First, health care professionals are not obliged to do that which violates their consciences or professional judgment. Second, distribution of limited resources to achieve fairness may override patient preferences. Third, social decisions about limiting the availability of certain forms of treatment and care may inhibit patient autonomy.

Commentary. Both the American social ethos and American law emphasize the primacy of individual choice. Health care, on the other hand, has traditionally favored paternalistic decision making by doctors for patients. There is now general consensus that competent patients are entitled to make their own decisions to accept or refuse treatment, even when their decisions could lead to earlier death.

Incompetent Patients

The President's Commission urges "health care professionals and institutions to "adopt clear, explicit, and publicly available policies regarding how and by whom decisions are to be made for patients who lack adequate decision-making capacity" (*Deciding to Forego,* pp. 5-6). They also prefer surrogate decision makers to use the substituted-judgment standard rather than the best-interests standard, except when insufficient information is available to make a substituted judgment. This means that for all patients who have *never* been competent, only the best-interests standard could be used.

Commentary. There is general consensus that incompetent patients ought not to be denied their right to make decisions simply because they are no longer able to express their preferences. Living wills, natural death act directives, patient-authorized do-not-resuscitate orders, uniform anatomical gift acts, and durable powers of attorney are all mechanisms devised to permit competent individuals to continue to direct their care even when they become incompetent. In many situations, however, patients have not made specific directives. When no one knows what the incompetent patient would have preferred, surrogate decision makers (usually family members) can make decisions. Whether or not these surrogate decision makers need to be legally appointed varies throughout the country.

There is no general agreement about what standard of judgment surrogate decision makers should use. Two standards are available: *substituted judgment* and *best interests. Substituted judgment* means that the surrogate attempts to decide what the specific person would have decided if he or she were able to do so, given that person's attitudes and values. It does *not* mean substituting the surrogate's judgment for the patient's. *Best interests,* on the other hand, attempts to balance the potential burdens and benefits of alternative forms of treatment and no treatment at all, thereby attempting to determine what most people would choose in that situation.

The best-interests standard can also be described as the kind of decision that we generally expect parents to make for their children. Best interests tends to be what is medically best. Thus, for example, if most people would choose a certain treatment, even though the prognosis were very poor (for example, chemotherapy for a form of cancer with a very poor survival rate), a surrogate decision maker would consent to that treatment if he or she were following a best-interests standard. If, on the other hand, the patient were someone who in his or her lifetime had avoided medical care, had religious beliefs about the undesirability of certain kinds of treatment, or had expressed desires about not being kept alive if incompetent, then the surrogate decision maker might

refuse the treatment on the basis of substituted judgment.

Similarly, if most people would refuse to continue ventilator support if they were permanently unconscious, then a surrogate making a best-interests decision in a similar case would choose to withdraw the respirator. If the patient had indicated, while competent, that he or she wanted everything done for him, then substituted judgment would demand a decision to continue ventilator support. A decision made on the basis of substituted judgment requires some explanation of what leads the decision maker to believe that the patient would have chosen the course under question.

Georgetown University philosopher Robert Veatch has argued that only surrogate decision makers who have personal and emotional ties to the patient should be permitted to make substituted judgments.[12] Decision makers without personal ties to the patient should, he argues, be restricted to the best-interests standard.[1]

Others, however, have argued that only legally authorized surrogate decision makers should be allowed to make substituted judgment decisions.

Permanently Unconscious Patients

The President's Commission believes that families should make the decision about continuing treatment for permanently unconscious patients and states that the law does not require *either* continuing *or* stopping treatment. The commission also discusses questions of providing specific forms of supportive care, including respirators, artificial feeding, dialysis, hygiene and skin care, and antibiotic treatment for infections (*Deciding to Forego,* pp. 190-191). With respect to providing food and fluids, the commission takes this position:

> Since permanently unconscious patients will never be aware of nutrition, the only benefit to the patient of providing such increasingly burdensome interventions [as artificial feeding] is sustaining the body to allow for a remote possibility of recovery. The sensitivities of the family and of care giving professionals ought to determine whether such interventions are made.

Commentary. Because permanently unconscious patients are not dead, it is generally considered appropriate to continue providing life-sustaining treatment if the surrogate decision makers judge that to be the best course to follow. There is, however, consensus that withdrawing life-sustaining treatment (but not withholding basic nursing care) is a morally appropriate course of action in some cases. In many cases, the decision focuses on removing the respirator from the permanently unconscious patient. In others, however, the focus may be on using antibiotics or providing food and fluids.

There is far more agreement about the appropriateness of withholding respirators than of withholding antibiotics; more agreement about the appropriateness of withholding antibiotics than of withholding food and fluids. The latter is, in particular, controversial. (Withholding food and fluids for patients who are conscious is discussed later in this chapter, but see also the case of *Claire Conroy,* chapter 14.)

Seriously Ill Patients

The President's Commission urges that competent patients and incompetent patients' surrogate decision makers be consulted about do-not-resuscitate orders for seriously ill patients. In the case of any disagreement between competent patient and physician, the patient should be transferred to a physician who is in agreement with the patient's preferences about the resuscitation order. In the case of any disagreement between the surrogate decision maker and the physician, the commission believes that the question should be submitted to institutional review and, if necessary, judicial review. The commission also emphasizes that a decision not to resuscitate holds "no necessary implications for any other therapeutic decisions" (*Deciding to Forego,* p. 251).

Commentary. There is general consensus that decisions not to resuscitate are appropriate in some cases in which resuscitating a patient may appear, on balance, to have fewer benefits than burdens. Of course, there is an inherent problem in knowing how to weigh benefits and burdens for individual patients. Many hospitals now have formal policies requiring that CPR always be performed unless there is a written do-not-resuscitate order. Furthermore, they require that competent patients and surrogate decision makers for incompetent patients consent to the writing of the order. However, strict adherence to these policies is not apparent and several studies show that consent is frequently not sought. In addition, there appears to be a high incidence of so-called slow codes and partial codes. This is likely to be an area of continuing controversy. Stuart Youngner, M.D., recently suggested that continued aggressive treatment of patients with written do-not-resuscitate orders may require some justification.[2] That is, although a DNR order has no *"necessary* implications for other thera-

peutic decisions," some decisions to treat may require justification. In light of continuing efforts to reduce hospital costs, especially for terminal care, treatment policies for DNR patients, with respect to the risk of both over-treatment and under-treatment, may need careful scrutiny by ethics committees.

Seriously Ill Newborns

The President's Commission sets the infant's best interests as the appropriate standard for treatment decisions for seriously ill newborns and affirms that no one is required to provide treatment that will be futile. By implication, at least, the commission acknowledges the legitimacy of quality-of-life considerations (although they do not use those words) when it states that "the concept of benefit necessarily makes reference to the context of the infant's present and future treatment, taking into account such matters as the level of biomedical knowledge and technology and the availability of services necessary for the child's treatment" (*Deciding to Forego,* p.7).

Commentary. The treatment of seriously ill newborns is the subject of recent federal legislation, the 1984 Amendments to the Child Abuse Prevention and Treatment Program Act,[3] which adopted standards that are not entirely consistent with the standards of the President's Commission. The federal legislation and accompanying regulations are intended to prohibit the use of quality-of-life considerations and appear to require that treatment be provided in almost all instances in which any life-saving benefit is possible. Exceptions include when the infant is permanently unconscious, when treatment would be virtually futile and inhumane, and when treatment will only prolong the dying process. The regulations do state that reasonable medical judgment is to be the standard for treatment decisions in these very difficult cases. The amendments were a response to the 1982 case in Indiana of an infant with Down's syndrome and esophageal atresia whose parents refused to consent to surgery to repair the atresia. Several physicians did not agree on what was the best course of treatment to take, and the Indiana courts supported the parents' right to choose between the two courses of medical treatment that had been recommended to them (to operate and not to operate). The law urges, but does not require, that infant care review committees be formed in hospitals with neonatal intensive care units and that these interdisciplinary committees review all cases prospectively in which treatment is to be foregone for a seriously ill newborn. The law uses the terms "infant care review committee" rather than "ethics committee" because it sees the committee's review function as that of ensuring that the standards contained within the regulation are adhered to. That is, the committee is not making independent ethical judgments about when treatment is appropriate. In that sense, the infant care review committees have something in common with the *Quinlan* prognosis committees.

Withholding Food and Fluids

The President's Commission believes that it is not necessary to continue feeding permanently unconscious patients if the family prefers not to do so, and that "only rarely should a dying patient be fed by tube or intravenously" *(Deciding to Forego,* p. 288). However, they do not address the question of providing food and fluids for the nondying, senile patient.

Commentary. There are many different kinds of patients who require artificial food and fluids, either because they can not or will not eat or because hand-feeding them is difficult. This group ranges from competent patients with no illness (individuals who pursue voluntary fasts for political reasons) to permanently unconscious patients (such as Karen Quinlan). It also includes competent patients with nonterminal illnesses (a fragile, elderly patient with a broken hip who will never recover mobility and wants to die quietly by declining food); competent patients with severe and irreversible physical disabilities who are no longer able to respond physically in a meaningful way to their surroundings (patients with amyotrophic lateral sclerosis or spinal cord injury); arguably competent patients with severe handicaps (such as Elizabeth Bouvia); terminally ill patients whose death is inevitable but not imminent (the final-stage cancer patient who repeatedly removes a nasogastric tube); patients with severe and irreversible dementia who have lost self-awareness but not consciousness (patients with advanced Alzheimer's disease); and bedridden, aged, and uncooperative patients with chronic mental illness or life-long severe retardation. The primary risk is that food and fluids will be withheld from patients because they are perceived to have little social value (the retarded, the demented, the isolated) or because their care is unrewarding, difficult, or expensive.

Although several court decisions have permitted the withdrawal of artificially supplied food and fluids from both conscious and unconscious patients, some courts have not. There continues to be considerable disagreement about the appropriateness of such actions. One disagreement focuses on whether providing food and fluids is "treatment" or "standard nursing care." Another more serious discussion focuses on the appropriateness of withholding food and fluids

when there is no terminal illness, because the patient would then die of starvation or dehydration. There is considerable fear that in these cases, decisions to withhold food and fluids may serve not the patient's interests but those of the care givers, of the family, or of society. Decisions to withhold food and fluids should always be very carefully considered.

Allocation of Resources

In *Securing Access to Health Care,* the President's Commission does not make specific recommendations regarding health care rationing. It does, however, suggest guidelines for ethical policies. These include "ensuring equitable access" to an adequate level of care for all citizens; obliging individuals with resources to pay a fair share of the costs; and widely distributing the burden of costs for those who cannot pay. The commission defines *adequate level of health care* as "enough care to achieve sufficient welfare, opportunity, information and evidence of interpersonal concern to facilitate a reasonably full and satisfying life" (p. 20). This may be less than *all beneficial care, all needed care,* or *all desired care.* The commission's view stresses the difference between *equity* and *equality:* some persons (those who can afford it) will be able to purchase much more health care service than others. That is not equal. Yet there is equity in that everyone has access to an adequate level of care; that is, a floor is set and no one need go beneath that level, though some will rise above it.

Commentary. The President's Commission does not argue that everyone has a moral right to health care but that society should provide access to everyone. There is, of course, no legally recognized right to health care. Because *rights* entail *duties,* if there were a right to health care, then someone would have a duty to provide that care. At this time, no such duty is legally recognized in the United States (except that owed to prisoners). There is, however, a constitutional duty not to discriminate (on the basis of race, handicap, religion, and so forth) whenever care is provided.

"Allocation of resources" refers to distribution processes. It does not imply any shortages. Thus, a hospital might allocate its nursing care so that everyone received what was needed. When allocation becomes rationing, it means that the resource supply is no longer adequate to meet the needs. Allocation is ordinarily the function of the hospital administration. However, when shortages develop and conscious decisions about rationing become necessary, ethics committees may become involved, insofar as rationing decisions usually imply ethical questions about just or fair distribution. It is not yet clear how—or if—ethics committees will be asked to respond to health care rationing.

Concerns about the effects of reduced health care spending are now being heard. Many have expressed fears or have cited instances of Medicare patients being discharged earlier than might be desirable, or even safe, because they have overstayed the number of diagnosis-related-group (DRG)-approved hospitalization days. Similarly, there are reports about denial of reimbursement for treatment of patients with DNR orders. There have been several well-documented instances of emergency care being denied to patients who were not insured or for whom insurance status information was unknown. Increased interest in permitting patients to refuse life-prolonging treatment is sometimes fueled by a desire to reduce end-of-life health care costs. Other areas in which rationing considerations are likely to arise include bed occupancy in intensive care units (for example, patients with DNR orders being kept out of ICU beds), distribution of the limited supply of transplant organs, and distribution of insufficient nursing services. Any situation in which care is provided and in which, at least in somebody's judgment, the care is not worth its cost (either the patient or society is not getting enough return on its investment) will provide an opportunity to consider rationing or reducing care.

In general, rationing decisions should be made not at the individual case level but at the policy level. The policy is then implemented in each individual case. Ethics committees will be most effective with respect to rationing by helping to develop policies that are sensitive to the ethical issues as well as responsive to the practical constraints that reduced resources necessitate. Of course, the primary problems come when ethical requirements conflict with practical constraints.

The coming years are likely to see continued financial constraints in health care because the cost of medical technology continues to rise dramatically.

That is, this problem (unlike disconnecting respirators from permanently unconscious patients or declaring death by brain-death criteria) will not be solved by some kind of consensus judgment. The problem will reassert itself with each new expensive medical development. It is possible that there will be increased emphasis on demonstrating the net effectiveness, the burdens and benefits, of new, complex forms of treatment before they are used. These demonstrations have generally been absent in the past, but if they become common, the ethics committee will find its role easier —it will have better information upon which to make its recommendations.

Notes

1. Veatch, R. Limits of guardian treatment refusal: A reasonableness standard. Am J Law Med. 1984. 9:427-68.

2. Youngner, S. Do-not-resuscitate orders: incidence and implications in a medical intensive care unit. *JAMA.* 1985. 253(1):54-7. See, also, Veatch, R. Deciding against resuscitations. *JAMA.*1985. 253(1):77-8.

3. *Federal Register.* 1985 Apr. 15. pp. 14878-901.

Reference

President's Commission for the Study of Ethical Problems in Medicine and Biomedical and Behavioral Research. *Defining Death,* 1981: *Whistleblowing in Biomedical Research,* 1981; *Compensating for Research Injuries,* 2 vols., 1982; *Protecting Human Subjects,* 1981; *Splicing Life,* 1982; *Making Health Care Decisions,* 3 vols., 1982-3; *Deciding to Forego Life-Sustaining Treatment,* 1983; *Implementing Human Research Regulations,* 1983; *Screening and Counselling for Genetic Conditions,* 1983; *Securing Access to Health Care,* 3 vols., 1983; and *Summing Up,* 1983. Washington, DC: U.S. Government Printing Office.

Chapter 4

A Process for Resolving Bioethical Dilemmas

An ethical dilemma arises when there is tension between loyalties, rights, duties, or values, all of which are good in themselves, but not all of which can be satisfied in a particular situation. Health care today presents many such dilemmas, largely because of our ability to sustain life. Sometimes the value of preserving life conflicts with other values, such as the value of respecting patients' wishes, the value of relieving suffering, the value of staying financially solvent, or the value of assuring equal access to health care for all. New and difficult questions face health professionals, patients, and families. When should do-not-resuscitate orders be written? Should an infant with microcephaly and other anomalies be treated? Is it ever right to withhold fluids and nutrition from a patient?

These and other questions require that a variety of factors—medical, ethical, legal, and interpersonal—be considered. The complexity of the issues suggests that a collaborative approach to resolving them will be more satisfactory than an individual or ad hoc method. However, for this collaboration to function effectively, it is necessary that the persons involved have some systematic approach to the process of working through an ethical dilemma. What follows is a process suggested for such an approach. It is developed primarily for use by ethics committees but may be helpful to anyone facing a bioethical dilemma.

The process involves four major steps. First, one must gather and assess the facts. Second, it is necessary to name the dilemma (that is, to specify the values that are in conflict) and establish the priorities among the relevant ethical principles. The third step is to consider alternative courses of action. The fourth step is to consider and decide upon implementation and follow-up. (This is not meant to imply that the committee is making patient care decisions, rather that it must do *something* with whatever conclusions it reaches in each case, even if that something is merely reporting its opinion to those who requested the case review.)

Gather and Assess the Facts

The first and most important step is to gather and assess the facts. For decisions about foregoing treatment, for example, the following questions may be relevant, although the list is not, of course, exclusive.

- Medical facts
  - What is the patient's current medical status?
  - Are there other contributing medical conditions?
  - What is the diagnosis? The prognosis? How reliable are these?
  - Has a second opinion been obtained? Would it be helpful?
  - Are there other tests that could help clarify the situation?
  - What treatments are possible?
  - What is the probable life expectancy and what will be the general condition if treatment is given?
  - What are the risks and side effects of treatment?
  - What is the probability that treatment will benefit the patient?
  - What benefits will treatment provide?
- Patient preference
  - Is the patient competent? That is, does he or she understand the need for medical care, the options that are available, and the probable results of choosing each of the various available courses of action?

- Has the patient been informed about his or her condition?
- How was the patient informed?
- Have all the treatment alternatives and their possible consequences been discussed with the patient?
- Has the patient had time to reflect upon the situation and upon the possible options?
- Has the patient made a clear statement about his or her wishes? If so, what are they?
- Has the patient discussed the situation thoroughly with someone other than the members of the immediate health care team?
- If the patient is not now competent, is he or she expected to regain competence?
- If the patient is incompetent, did he or she ever make a clear statement that would indicate what his or her wishes would be in these circumstances?
- Has the patient prepared a written statement regarding his or her wishes?
- Has the patient signed a durable power of attorney for health care? A living will? A natural death act?
- How physically and emotionally healthy was the patient before this current situation?
- If the patient has made no clear statement, is there information from anyone regarding what the patient might have wanted or might reasonably be assumed to have wanted?
- Views of family and friends
  - Are there family members and/or friends? Who are they?
  - Do they fully understand the patient's condition?
  - What are their positions?
  - Do they agree with one another?
  - Are there any reasons to question their motives?
  - Has one person been identified as having the primary responsibility for communication and decision making?
  - Does anyone have legal custody of the patient (guardianship or conservatorship)?
  - If the patient is a minor and the parent(s) are the legal guardians, are they choosing a course of action that is clearly in the child's best interests?
  - If there are problems in communicating with family and/or friends, can someone be found (a minister, for example) who could be helpful?
- Views of the care givers
  When the ethics committee is asked to review a case, the chairman should invite the primary care givers to be present for the discussion. In addition to physicians, this might include nurses, social workers, and chaplains.
  - Are the care givers fully apprised of the facts?
  - What are their views?
  - Why do they hold those views?
  - If the care givers disagree, what accounts for the disagreements? Can they be resolved?
- Legal, administrative, and external factors
  - Are there state statutes or case law that apply to this situation?
  - What potential liability might be present with respect to the hospital, to the providers, and to the parent or guardian?
  - Are there hospital policies or guidelines that apply?
  - Are there other persons (in or outside the institution) who should be given information or asked for an opinion?
  - Would it help to consult the literature for any aspect of this case?
  - Is expense to the patient and/or family a factor in this case?

Name the Dilemma

Naming the dilemma involves identifying the values in conflict. If they are not *ethical* values or principles, it is not truly an ethical dilemma. It may be a communication problem or an administrative or legal uncertainty. The values, rights, duties, or ethical principles in conflict should be evident and the dilemma should be named as in this example: "This is a case of conflict between patient autonomy and doing good for the patient." When these principles come into conflict, a choice will have to be made about which principles should be preserved. The committee should clearly articulate why that choice is made. The ethical principles most frequently involved in these situations are discussed more fully in "Ethical Principles in Health Care," in chapter 2. They include:

- *Patient autonomy.* If the competent patient has made a clear statement regarding his or her wishes, the patient's autonomy—the right to self-determination or freedom of choice—should be respected. (Some rare exceptions occur, as in the case of a patient wanting the hospital to assist with a suicide or in the case of a patient demanding medically inappropriate, unreasonable treatment.) Full information must be given to the patient in order for freedom of choice to be possible, unless the patient states that he or she does not want it.

- *Beneficence.* Doing good for others; considerate, respectful, and compassionate care.
- *Nonmaleficence.* Doing no harm. The person should never be directly harmed or treated as if he or she were merely the means to an end.
- *Justice.* People in similar situations should be treated similarly. They should not be discriminated against on the basis of such factors as mental ability or social contribution.
- *Truth-telling.* Honesty or integrity.
- *Promise-keeping.* Honoring of a covenant; fidelity.

Alternative Courses of Action

When faced with a difficult dilemma, individuals often see only two courses of action. In reality, there are frequently many alternative courses of action that can be explored. These may relate to choosing treatment, to dealing with family and friends, or to exploring available resources. It is good to brainstorm about all the possible actions that could be taken, even if some have already been informally excluded. This process gives everyone a chance to think through the possibilities and to make clear arguments for and against the various alternatives. It also helps to discourage any possible polarization of the parties involved.

Implementation and Follow-up

Ordinarily, the members of the ethics committee and the other participants will arrive at a consensus about the best resolution of the dilemma or about acceptable options. Even if there is disagreement about the most appropriate course of action, *some conclusion* will have been reached about what steps are appropriate. It should be made clear to the members of the group what conclusions have been reached and what will be done with that information. These and other questions should be asked: What steps, if any, will be taken next? By whom? How should the discussion and the conclusions be communicated to the interested parties who have not participated in the discussion? Is there a process to handle any remaining concerns of the principal parties? Did issues arise that could be discussed in an educational session for the hospital staff? Are policies or guidelines needed to address similar situations? What can be learned from this experience?

References

Aroskar, M. Anatomy of an ethical dilemma: the theory. *Am J Nursing.* 1980. 80(4):658-63.

Holmes, C. Bioethical decision making: an approach to improve the process. *Med Care.* 1979. 17(1):1131-8.

Jonsen, A. E., Siegler, M., and Winslade, W. J. *Clinical Ethics.* New York: Mcmillan Co., 1982.

Purtillo, R. B., and Cassel, C. K. *Ethical Dimensions in the Health Professions.* Philadelphia: W. B. Saunders, 1981, pp. 25-9, 210-2.

Siegler, M. Decision making strategy for clinical-ethical problems in medicine. *Arch Intern Med.* 1982. 14(12):2178-9.

Swazey, J. P. To treat or not to treat: the search for principled decisions. In: Abernethy, V., ed. *Frontiers in Medical Ethics: Applications in a Clinical Setting.* Cambridge, MA: Ballinger, 1980, pp. 139-55.

Part **II**

Bioethics Committees in Practice

Chapter 5

Committee Structure

Until very recently, hospital ethics committees had been created in response to a specific need perceived by the hospital community. Now, many committees are being created in the wake of the Baby Doe regulations and the subsequent 1984 Amendments to the Child Abuse Prevention and Treatment Program Act, which focused considerable attention on ethics committees. Whereas the legislation does not require the formation of ethics committees (and, in fact, the regulations accompanying the legislation specifically deny the use of the term "ethics" in referring to infant care review committees), a hospital ought to be very sure that it knows why it needs an ethics committee before deciding to start one. This chapter examines the practical issues that should be considered in establishing an ethics committee.

Getting Started

In our experience, most committees have been started as a result of one or two health professionals feeling particularly disturbed about difficulties in making decisions regarding termination of dialysis treatment, withdrawal of a respirator, or another specific issue. Whatever the focus, there should be some specific question, some specific need, some specific problem to which the committee can respond. Sometimes this question or problem is fully articulated: "We need a policy on withdrawing respirators." Other times, it is a much more vaguely expressed need: "We have a problem about withdrawing respirators because there's a lot of disagreement about what is going on and we don't know how to handle it." Before an individual or a group embarks on an ethics committee, they should be able to give at least a tentative answer to the question: What are this hospital's specific needs with regard to ethical issues in health care and why is a committee needed to fulfill them?

Given the hierarchical structure of the hospital, it might appear that only physicians could initiate such a committee. However, in our experience, it is evident that the initial actions can be taken by anyone: nurse, social worker, respiratory therapist, administrator, chaplain, or physician. For a committee to be successful over time, it must be multidisciplinary and it must have support from both the physicians and the hospital administration, but at the beginning it needs only the interest and energies of someone or some small group. It is the first responsibility of that individual or small group to gather some official backing. The group must read the atmosphere of their individual hospital to determine whether administrative or medical support should be sought first. Ultimately, both are needed, but approaching these two groups involves assessing the politics of the individual hospital.

In order to gain official support, the initiating group must have some clear sense of what such a committee has to offer the hospital. The group might want to prepare a list of paradigmatic or actual cases that have provoked problems in the past, or to list specific kinds of inconsistencies in treatment decisions that have led to staff morale problems. In some way, the group should be able to document a genuine set of problems that needs to be addressed. It need not be exhaustive and it need not involve consultation and case review, but it does need to be real.

When official backing has been gathered and a decision to proceed has been made (this may imply some kind of official support or it may involve only tacit approval), at least three possible directions can be followed. First, a task force may be appointed to assess the need for an ethics committee. Second, a bioethics study group may be formed to enable the interested parties to increase their understanding of the issues. And third, a bioethics committee may be formed to undertake any or all of the possible functions of the committee.

Although it has not been customary to start with a task force, we believe that this is the preferable way to begin. Official appointment of a task force gives authoritative sanction to the possibility of an ethics committee. The task force can determine if there is a realistic need for an ethics committee as well as a realistic possibility of its being able to function effectively in that particular hospital. If the task force finds that a committee would be advisable, it should also make recommendations about the committee's goals, functions, and place in the organizational structure. The task force may then form the core of the ethics committee, although it need not. (Those who are in a good position to assess the hospital's needs may not be the best persons to serve on an ethics committee.)

A committee that arises from task force deliberations should begin life with some degree of structure. Its members will probably have been appointed deliberately to achieve specific distribution balance (for example, equal numbers of physicians, nurses, and others). It should have a written statement of its functions and goals. It should have some kind of financial and clerical support.

When a committee begins as a study group or as an ad hoc ethics committee, it will (and should) have much less structure. Members are often volunteers, terms of office are undetermined, and official support may be uncertain. Such a group ought not be too concerned initially about providing structures or defining specific procedures for the group to follow. As it develops, the group will begin to sense how it can best serve the hospital community. Until then, however, it should probably remain informal in as many aspects as possible. It is likely to have a considerable degree of momentum when it forms, and to use up that energy in discussing questions of committee structure too soon will be counterproductive and diversionary. It is easy for everyone to get caught up in time-consuming structural questions because they are so much more familiar and so much easier to think about than the substantive questions of bioethics or the political problems that can affect the ethics com-

mittee. Just because of that, it is wise to postpone the structural questions for as long as possible.

Taking a slow approach may not be possible, however, if the committee is created by official action without an intervening task force committee and is expected to begin functioning formally in reasonably short order. Even then, however, it would be well to make as few structural decisions as possible. Later on, when they see how the committee is actually functioning in the hospital, the members will have a much better sense of how the whole thing can be best constructed. If some decisions do need to be made, the characteristics of the individual hospital should be considered. For example, in deciding the number of members needed, it might be advisable to consider whether this is a hospital in which people generally attend meetings or one in which they frequently do not attend meetings. If attendance is going to be a problem (and it is in many hospitals), then a larger committee may be necessary in order to ensure a large enough group for each meeting.

Defining Goals and Functions

A wide range of ethical issues might be under the committee's purview, including clinical care issues, patient advocacy concerns, the problems of impaired physicians and nurses, the implementation of philosophy in religious hospitals, and conflicts generated by physician joint ventures. Of course, a committee may choose to address any of these issues that are within its general mandate. For the most part, however, time is so short that most ethics committees choose to address themselves exclusively to bioethical and clinical care problems. Other problems, although they involve important ethical issues, may be better dealt with by other hospital committees and the ethics committee will probably do better work by narrowing its scope. Robert Veatch, a philosopher at the Kennedy Institute of Ethics, Georgetown University, Washington, DC, has suggested that allocation issues, clinical care issues, and patient advocacy issues might all require separate ethics committees because the underlying principles of each would differ substantially.[1] Whatever issues a committee chooses to deal with, the members should delineate their goals in terms of the scope of those ethical issues and should be certain that they have the appropriate membership on the committee for dealing with those issues.

The committee should have or should write a statement of its functions. The three standard functions of ethics committees are education (of the committee members, of the hospital physicians and staff members, of patients and families, and of the local hospital community); policy recommendation (policies and guidelines for health care professionals regarding decision-making processes in problematic cases and for allocation issues); and case review (prospective and retrospective review). The statement of the committee's functions should be detailed rather than perfunctory, explaining both why the committee has chosen these functions and how it intends to carry them out. The writing of this statement will require the committee members to consider seriously what they can reasonably do and to establish effective priorities for use of time. Without such a statement, there is a very high probability of dissipation of efforts over too wide a field. (Samples of committee "statements of function" are included in appendix B.)

In some instances, it becomes apparent when writing a committee function statement that there is too much work for the committee to do. This suggests the need for more than one committee. Especially when there are recurring issues that require a considerable investment of time, it may be appropriate either to appoint a permanent subcommittee or to create a separate committee. In many hospitals, the significant problems involving critically ill newborns have led either to separate committees or to subcommittees addressing infant care issues. Even when the committees are separate, they sometimes have overlapping membership. The regulations implementing the 1984 Amendments to the Child Abuse Prevention and Treatment Program Act recommend separate infant care review committees. The regulations choose not to call these committees ethics committees because their primary responsibility is assessing treatment decisions as medical decisions, not as ethical decisions. (In that sense, these DHHS-recommended committees may be more like the prognosis committees recommended by the New Jersey Supreme Court in the *Karen Quinlan* case.) Neonatal committees may, of course, address ethical issues, just as more general ethics committees do.

Hospitals that provide experimental treatments (for example, bone marrow transplant or other organ transplants that are seen as experimental) may want to have separate committees to deal specifically with ethical problems that arise with each type of treatment and are not addressed by institutional review boards. Similarly, very large hospitals may find that issues frequently arise in dialysis units or intensive care units and that a specific committee is needed to address these issues. On the other hand, for most hospitals a single ethics committee will suffice.

The committee should establish realistic goals and should review them regularly (at least every six months). Articulating goals, like delineating functions, means that priorities must be set and limits acknowledged. For the most part, committees take on too much, too quickly. A newly formed committee that seriously expects to educate itself and the hospital community, to make policy recommendations, and to provide case review, all within the first year, is probably taking on too much—unless the hospital's support for the committee's work is very strong and the committee members' experience and background with bioethical issues is considerable.

Organizational Placement

At some point (depending upon how the committee gets started), someone will have to decide where an ethics committee best fits in the hospital organizational structure. An ethics committee can be constituted as a medical staff committee, as an administrative committee, or as a governing board committee. Most committees have been formed as either medical staff committees or as administrative committees. Board committees remain relatively rare.

Organizational placement may affect three different concerns: the discoverability of committee records; the specific membership on the committee, the manner of appointing members, and the selection of the committee chairman; and the character of the committee. The currently high number of medical staff committees appears to be a result of concern about the discoverability of committee records.

Discoverability

Although state laws differ on the issue of discoverability, many states provide immunity for the records of hospital committees whose function it is to oversee and take steps to improve overall patient care. Utilization review and quality assurance committees are paradigms of that kind of committee. The reader is advised to consult an attorney familiar with the laws of his or her state for specific information on this question. The relevant California statute (Evidence Code, section 1157) reads, in part:

> Neither the proceedings nor the records of organized committees of medical . . . staffs in hospitals having the responsibility of evaluation and improvement in the quality of care rendered in the hospital . . . shall be subject to discovery.

As a matter of public policy, states may take the position that the hospital committee's ability to act freely to investigate and correct patient care problems is more important than the court's having access to the committee's records, even through subpoena. If a state has chosen to protect the records of such hospital committees, which are customarily medical staff committees, then it may choose to extend that protection to ethics committees. There is considerable controversy about whether or not ethics committees fill the same type of role as, for example, quality assurance committees and about whether their records would be protected in the event of suit, even if the committee were constituted as a medical staff committee. Nevertheless, the likelihood of committee records being nondiscoverable is greater if the committee is a medical staff committee rather than an administrative or board committee.

It should be noted that some have claimed that when a chart note refers to ethics committee review, all committee records relevant to that case would be discoverable. Other legal writers have disputed this claim. The fact is that ethics committees are so new that no one really knows how the law will handle them. As of this writing, there has been no case involving ethics committees and their records, so we have no case law for guidance.

A second matter related to discoverability is whether or not committee members can be subpoenaed to testify about what went on at meetings. Some individuals have stated that if the committee's records are not discoverable, members who attended meetings cannot be required to testify about what transpired at a meeting. This is not entirely correct: California's statute, for example, allows testimony about "statements made by any person in attendance at such a meeting who is a party to an action or proceeding the subject matter of which was reviewed at such meeting." There are other exceptions involving testimony, as well.

The relationships between discoverability, accountability, and confidentiality are discussed further in chapter 11, "Privacy, Confidentiality, and Privilege." Committees should give serious consideration to the importance of discoverability. Many committees assume that protecting committee records is of vital importance. They should be aware that there is no consensus on this issue and that many commentators believe that because the public approval for ethics committees arises from a desire for public accountability in regard to difficult legal and ethical health care decisions, an aura of or a desire for secrecy is highly inappropriate. If the committee records are written to preserve confidentiality, then concerns about what would happen if they were made public in legal proceedings may have very little substance.

Membership Requirements and Selection

Medical staff committees typically require that at least half the members be medical doctors. Governing board committees may require that some number of the trustees be members of the committee. Administrative committees typically have no requirements about membership. From the perspective of ensuring multidisciplinary membership, the administrative committee is the best form. However, even though a medical staff committee needs to "look like" a medical staff committee (that is, include a substantial number of medical staff members, be incorporated into the medical staff bylaws, and be responsible to the executive committee of the medical staff), such a committee can certainly include a substantial number of nonphysicians and thus encompass a multidisciplinary membership. It may be somewhat more difficult for a board committee to be truly multidisciplinary without going outside the board for its membership, but some board committees have been effectively organized to accommodate this need.

The three types of committees differ with respect to who actually appoints the members (namely a medical executive committee, the administration, or the governing board); however, there is no reason to suppose that a competent and representative group of people cannot be chosen.

The chairman of a medical staff committee is customarily a physician. Administrative or board committees may be chaired by physicians but are sometimes chaired by other professionals. Although some have argued that an ethics committee will lack credibility without a physician as its chairman, the existence of many effective and credible ethics committees with nurses, administrators, chaplains, or social workers as chairmen or cochairmen makes that an empty claim. Credibility is a problem if there are not enough physicians on the committee, but physicians need not chair the committee. Many committees have cochairmen, one a physician, the other a nurse, social worker, or pastoral care representative.

Character of the Committee

The type of ethics committee that a hospital chooses to establish can make various statements about the committee's role. An administrative or board committee gives the clear message that ethical concerns are not solely or primarily medical questions, of interest only to the medical staff. An administrative or board committee may also give greater acknowledgment to the equal status of all members of the committee, each drawing upon his or her unique expertise. Such a committee is a model of the interdisciplinary collaboration that can occur throughout the hospital. A medical staff committee may also be able to achieve this democratic character, but medical staff committees are more likely to reinforce rather than to minimize a hospital's hierarchical structure. Furthermore, a medical staff committee may suggest that the issues are primarily medical.

Note

1. Veatch, R. Hospital ethics committees: is there a role? *Hastings Cent Rep.* 1977. 7:22-5.

References

Fost, N., and Cranford, R. E. Hospital ethics committees: administrative aspects. *JAMA.* 1985. 253(918):2687-92.

Monagle, J.F. Blueprints for hospital ethics committees. *CHA Insight.* 1984. 8(20):1-4..

Robertson, J. A. Ethics committees in hospitals: Alternative structures and responsibilities. *QRB.* 1984 Jan. 10(1):6-10.

Veatch, R. M. Hospital ethics committees: is there a role? *Hasting Cent Rep.* 1977. 7(3):22-5.

Chapter 6

Committee Membership

The size of ethics committees varies widely, sometimes as a function of the committees' origins. On the one hand, groups that began as bioethics study groups and slowly evolved into ethics committees tend to keep all participants as members of the committee. In some instances, this means a committee of 25 or more. On the other hand, committees that formed specifically as ethics committees are likely to be smaller, with 12 to 15 members, although some have as few as 8 members. There is no perfect size for a committee, though a good deal of unproductive time can be spent pondering the question.

As is true with regard to many choices that need to be made, *a clear idea of the committee's function will help to resolve the question of size.* If the committee's role is primarily educational, then a large group may well be appropriate and preferable. If the committee intends to conduct "whole-committee" case reviews, then 25 is probably too large to permit serious participation by all members. (New England communities, which conduct large town meetings very effectively, show that considerable skill and extremely good planning is necessary to ensure sensitive and thoughtful consideration of an issue in a large group.) If the committee plans to focus on writing policies, then a medium-size group may be best. If the committee plans to do all three, then it may help to have a larger group in order to handle the large amount of work, primarily through subcommittees. The hospital may have many people interested in becoming members, or very few. This, too, will affect size: better to have a small, interested group than a large indifferent one.

Who are the members? This question actually holds within it two other questions. Those forming an ethics committee or recruiting new members need to ask not only what kind of backgrounds the members should have, but also what kind of persons they should be. Too frequently the question of title is mulled over extensively with little or no consideration given to the question of the nature, the character, or the attitude of prospective members. We believe that personal qualities—that is, attitudes, temperament, and the capacity for critical thinking—are more important than educational field or degrees. To ensure diversity and to be fair, the committee should be generally representative of the hospital community, but the most exquisitely representative committee will do no good if its members are not thoughtful, reflective, critical thinkers who are willing and able to move slowly, to tolerate substantial ambiguity, and to accept and respect one another.

The Kind of Person

It might seem that any interested health care professional would be a good member of an ethics committee. Some aspects of ethics committee work, however, require special attributes. Ethical analysis requires a problem-solving approach that is primarily reflective. Although many health care workers are thoughtful, reflective thinkers, clinical care does not primarily attract persons with that approach to problem solving, for good reason: hospitals are places in which the dominant mode is action. In hospitals, the physicians and staff are required to solve problems actively and quickly. Those who want to stop and think for a while, considering fully the pros and cons of a decision, would not last long in the hospital environment. Thus, for example, an exceptional ability to act with certainty and to make decisions quickly, even in the face of necessarily inadequate information, might mark a superb physician but not, necessarily, a good ethics committee member. Ethics committee members need to be open to different ideas. They need to be able to put aside their own judgments while they assess the logic and reasoning of those with different and perhaps unappealing values.

In addition, they need a fair degree of humility and both the willingness and the ability to work cooperatively with people who come from different levels within the hospital hierarchy. The fact that hospitals have such well-ingrained hierarchies creates a special problem in establishing ethics committees. Physicians who are willing to listen only to other physicians will be as counterproductive on an ethics committee as nurses who are willing to say what is on their minds only to other nurses. The ethics committee must function as a group of equals and members should be chosen for their ability to accept that equality.

Members need not be well-versed in ethics or the humanities, but they should be interested in learning about them, as opposed to being interested in imposing their own values on others. They should have the habit of thinking about right and wrong, even if not formally schooled in it. They should be willing to spend the extra time that will be needed to learn something that is distinct from medicine and patient care. One reason ethics committees are being formed at this time is that technical medical knowledge is not sufficient to answer the dilemmas that health care choices now pose. Committee members should not be so committed to science and medicine that they cannot imagine the validity of other perceptions of the world and of other ways of reaching answers to questions. The scientific method has provided extraordinary progress, but it is of little or no use in assessing problems about personal or social values. Thus, although most potential committee members will have been trained in science and the scientific method, they should be willing and able to move outside that frame of reference and to understand how the language and logic of ethics differ from those of science.

Potential members should be critical thinkers, able to follow an idea logically, and should possess sufficient discipline or patience to contemplate a problem before moving to an answer. Critical thinking implies a questioning attitude toward easy and even obvious answers without being disputatious or adversarial. Critical thinking enables a person to consider a problem in its immediate context and not to lose sight of the broader societal context that shapes the individual event in the present and will be shaped by individual events in the future. Critical thinkers always assume that there is more to a situation than meets the eye. Sometimes they are wrong; with respect to ethical issues in health care, they are usually right. Their insistence upon looking at other sides of the question may appear inefficient, but it is vital.

We do not intend this description of desirable qualities in ethics committee members to be too demanding, suggesting that only specially or highly educated people have these skills, or that only a few people have them. They are abilities possessed by many people in ordinary walks of life. The people who have these abilities may or may not currently be using them to think about ethical issues in health care. Once selected for ethics committee membership, they will be able to learn the relevant information and to apply their skills to the work of the committee.

Professional Backgrounds

Those who select ethics committee members may want to consider each potential member's professional and educational background. Or they may decide that any concerned hospital physician or staff member should be a member. Ethics committees that begin as study groups usually are happy to include everyone who is interested in the issue, even if the group's demography does not match that of the hospital itself. When members are specifically selected, they are sometimes chosen democratically, or sometimes drawn exclusively from the upper echelons of the hospital community. The latter method provides an authoritative but probably overly administrative committee, and its members may be too distant from the day-to-day activities of health care.

Committees that are formed by the medical executive committee frequently acquire half their members from the medical staff and draw the remaining half from hospital nurses, social workers, pastoral care representatives, and administrative staff. Other committees may have a smaller proportion of doctors and correspondingly more nurses, social workers, and clergy. We believe that a suitable composition for an ethics committee is one-third physicians; one-third nurses; and one-third others, including social workers, chaplains, administrators, nonhospital specialists (attorney, ethicist), and lay members. Nursing staff members should not be limited to nursing administrators, but should include staff nurses.

The committee may also include members from outside the hospital. These members might include an attorney (other than the hospital attorney) who is interested in health care; a philosopher or theologian (frequently recruited from neighboring colleges or universities); disabled adults, members of disability groups, or parents of disabled children (especially on committees addressing questions of treatment of handicapped newborns); clergy; and lay members representing community values.

Representativeness

For an ethics committee to gain credibility within the hospital and to provide accountability outside the hospital, it should be representative. (A nonrepresentative committee might do excellent work, but the work might not be perceived as excellent because of political concerns.) A committee composed only of physicians would probably lack sufficiently varied perspectives to respond to ethical dilemmas. Furthermore, if the public or the hospital community felt that the ethical conflicts of health care were adequately handled by physicians alone, the intense discussions about biomedical ethics during the past 15 years would not have taken place. Likewise, a committee that functioned without physicians would be equally inadequate. It would lack credibility, both within and without the hospital, because the physician's scientific and technologic knowledge and the relationship between doctor and patient are vital factors in identifying and resolving the bioethics dilemma. As noted, many committees give half their membership slots to physicians.

Other committees, however, are able to function successfully with a smaller proportion of physicians among their membership. Such committees should call upon specialists within the hospital whenever the committee lacks particular medical expertise. Each hospital should consider how representative its own committee needs to be in order to respond to the hospital's psychological and political demands. It should be noted, however, that if an ethics committee includes case review as its function, the committee should consider including members (doctors and nurses) from the NICU, the ICU, and other hospital units in which ethical problems arise frequently, because their clinical expertise will be needed by the committee.

Lawyers

Committees are frequently advised to include among their members a lawyer who is not a hospital employee. A person who is familiar with legal requirements and restrictions will be of vital importance to the committee, even if it does not conduct case reviews. The committee will need to keep abreast of legal developments in the field, and this too is a specialized field of study. (See chapters 10 through 14 for a layperson's guide to the legal system.) A lawyer serves the same kind of *professional* function on the committee as does a physician: he or she brings expert knowledge that the committee members need. Nonhospital lawyers are preferred, not because they are better lawyers or know more about ethics, but because the hospital lawyer is employed to protect the hospital's interests. Insofar as, in some cases, the hospital's interests (in avoiding possible law suits, for example) may not in the short run be consistent with the patient's desires or interests, the hospital lawyer should not to be placed in a position of possible conflict of interest. Certainly individual hospital lawyers are able to identify such conflicts of interest when they occur, but the committee members cannot be sure that will happen, and the hospital lawyer ought not to be asked to wear two hats at once.

If a lawyer is sought for committee membership because of the need for expertise, then it behooves the committee to find a person who has the specific expertise that is needed. An attorney brings to the committee a generalized skill in legal analysis. Beyond that, attorneys are, for the most part, just as specialized as physicians, although the legal profession generally lacks procedures for what would be comparable to formal board certification. It is certainly possible that any lawyer, including a retired or sitting judge, can be an excellent member, but it would help to have one who does not have to learn the legal background needed by the committee.

If the hospital is located near a law school, ethics committee members could inquire about any faculty member who has a particular interest or expertise in medical law. The local bar association may well have committees that deal with ethics, with medico-legal problems, or with bioethics issues. Ideally, the committee would be able to choose from among several qualified persons. Like all professionals, lawyers have personal values as well as professional ones, and the individual chosen should be someone with whom the other committee members feel comfortable, someone they can respect for the personal qualities of mind that he or she brings to the committee in addition to legal expertise. In addition, the lawyer chosen should understand that the committee's primary focus is on ethics, not law, though legal knowledge is an important component. Knowing what the law says about a topic does not end the discussion.

Ethicists

The bioethics movement has led to the creation of a new title: bioethicist. The bioethicist specializes in what might be called "applied ethics." Bioethicists are usually—but not always—theologians or philosophers who have studied and written about the moral implications and ethical nature of health care decisions, either at the policy level or in the clinical setting. Some bioethicists have degrees in law rather than philosophy or moral theology. The bioethicist's area of expertise is philosophical analysis of health care decisions that involve ethical conflicts. Most ethicists are university or college faculty members, usually associated with the school's department of philosophy, a religious studies program, or an interdisciplinary program that pursues studies in law, medicine, and philosophy. With increasing frequency, however, ethicists are found as full-time employees or part-time consultants in hospitals (especially teaching hospitals associated with medical schools and universities) or in hospital systems (especially Roman Catholic systems) throughout the country.

To urge that an ethics committee have among its members an ethicist is not to imply that the hospital has in its employ a full-time practitioner of applied ethics. Rather, it is to suggest that the committee find someone who has some professional skill in ethical analysis and who is willing to put these skills at the service of the committee. The theologian-philosopher who fills this "ethicist" role is not intended to provide "expert" moral judgments for the committee. The members, individually and as a group, must do this themselves. The ethicist's contribution (regardless of the committee's function) is to be sensitive to the committee's need for clarity, consistency, and principled reasoning. Although all committee members need to learn how to think consciously within an ethical frame of reference, the committee ethicist can help to get that process started and can provide a running check over time.

Some health care professionals feel that an ethicist is ultimately not helpful because he or she lacks an understanding of the clinical setting. Others, however, have pointed out that the ethicist's professional training in thinking things over without *having* to make a decision is an important attribute, because it balances medical training's heavy emphasis on active intervention. In addition, an ethicist brings to the committee a nonhospital perspective. Working in any institution over time places blinders on the employee. For the most part, people become accustomed to "how things are done here," regardless of where here is. The ethicist who comes from beyond the hospital walls may be able to broaden the committee members' views because his or her perspective differs from theirs (although, of course, it may have been correspondingly narrowed by some other institution).

If an ethics committee wishes to have an ethicist as a member, it will probably have to go out and find one. Local colleges or universities should be contacted. The committee might start by inquiring of the philosophy or theology department whether any faculty members have specialized in medical ethics, moral theology, bioethics, or applied ethics. The department will inevitably teach courses in ethics and, if no one specializes in medical ethics, the instructor of the ethics course can be asked if he or she knows of anyone in the vicinity who has specialized in medical ethics. The Society for Health and Human Values includes among its members philosophers, academicians from the fields of literature and history, theologians, physicians, and attorneys who are deeply interested in these matters. The society publishes a state-by-state membership list that might provide leads for the committee.

The committee may not need an ethicist if it has a health care professional who has done work in this area. Increasingly, physicians, nurses, and other health care professionals are taking individual bioethics courses, as well as fellowships and sabbaticals, that permit extended study of the relationship between medicine and ethics. Summer courses sponsored by the National Endowment for the Humanities; courses at the Kennedy Institute; sabbatical and degree study at the Institute for Medical Humanities at the Texas Medical Branch, Galveston; university extension courses; and other such courses may provide excellent background for the health care professional to take the part of the ethicist. The individual who has pursued the study of medical ethics should, however, be asked to decide if his or her knowledge is sufficient to fulfill this role.

Finding an ethicist might be some work for the committee, and the members may decide to get along without one, either because they do not know anyone who is qualified or because they have vague feelings that they do not need such a person to carry out the committee's work. Most health care providers feel perfectly competent in matters of morality, and some feel that calling in an "ethical specialist" suggests that they themselves are either ethically incompetent or actually unethical. This attitude results from a confusion between moral judgments and ethical arguments. It cannot be emphasized too strongly that the ethicist's role is to help the committee maintain standards of ethical analysis, not to provide moral judgments.

Lay Members

Ethics committees are frequently advised to include lay members in their number. Lay members are expected, it is usually said, either to provide "community values" or to ensure community credibility. In getting organized, a committee may have its hands full getting its hospital members together (and finding a nonhospital lawyer and ethicist). Institutional review boards are required to include lay members and the faint parallel between IRBs and ethics committees may account for this insistence upon lay membership. However, the committees are not exact parallels in this respect, and the arguments that make lay members very important to an IRB do not apply in the same way to an ethics committee. The question of lay membership on ethics committees is complex and one that can (and perhaps should) be postponed until the committee understands its function well enough to decide how lay members might help. There is no point in having lay members just to have them: they are not good-luck charms.

If and when the ethics committee decides to have lay members, it must understand why it wants them and what is meant by the word *lay*. A lay member might simply be someone who lives in the community served by the hospital. Thus, one southern California hospital ethics committee that serves a primarily Latino population, but whose staff and physicians are primarily white and black, has a Latino lay member. Similarly, a hospital with a substantial percentage of elderly patients or welfare patients might include as lay members one or more of its elderly or impoverished community members. Lay members might be those with a personal but nonmedical understanding of the medical problems that the committee considers. Thus, an infant care review committee might include as a lay member the parent of a handicapped child, a member of a handicapped persons' association, or an adult handicapped person.

Lay members might simply be thought of as those who are not health care professionals (in which case, the nonhospital lawyer and the ethicist could be considered lay members). Lay members might be those who neither work in the hospital nor hold professional credentials. A local real estate salesperson would fit that category. The Latino woman, the welfare recipient, the senior citizen, the paraplegic, the health-law attorney, and the real estate agent all have in common that they are not health care providers. They may have very little else in common, and the ethics committee should be very certain about the reasons for including such lay persons on the committee. Each would bring different skills and information to the committee.

When the committee members know what they are lacking, they can find the lay member they need. As with the selection of all members, when choosing a lay member the committee should be concerned with whether or not the person has the temperament and the time for committee work and for reflective analysis. Individuals might, for example, identify so strongly with their own views, or with those of the group they represent, that they cannot tolerate the views of others. The idea is not to have people representing special interests but to have people with special interests and skills joining with the committee in its work.

Some may charge that the ethics committee will not be sensitive to community values or will lack credibility in the community if there are no lay members. Several replies might be made to this contention. First, there is no reason to suppose that those in the hospital are insensitive to community values simply because they do not belong to the same ethnic group, share the same socioeconomic status, belong to the same age group, or live in the same neighborhood. The capacity for empathy and imagination lies within everyone and is exercised on more than rare occasions.

Second, it is not clear why the hospital should automatically accede to community values. If a Catholic hospital serves a community that is largely non-Catholic, it need not provide ordinary abortion services merely because abortion is consistent with community values. In addition, a hospital serving an upwardly mobile, middle-class population that has strong views about "quality of life," particularly with respect to mental disability, need not withhold treatment from any infant who might be retarded merely to serve community values.

Third, the community is seldom aware of hospital practices unless its citizens read about them in the newspaper. By and large, hospitals have great credibility within their communities. If a hospital has lost its credibility, placing a lay member on the ethics committee will not restore it. If a hospital has been involved in a case that has received widespread, critical publicity or has what is euphemistically known as a "public-relations problem," then a lay member may be an important consideration, but certainly not a solution to its problem. If the hospital is widely believed *not* to be protecting patients, then it has problems greater than an ethics committee can hope to solve.

An ethics committee that chooses to have a lay member should seriously consider having at least two lay members, especially if the committee is choosing community nonprofessionals. Many persons are intimidated by hospitals, by physicians, and by strangers. As a group of one, the lay member may be too inclined to defer to the larger group. Certainly there is a very great risk of the single lay member being immediately coopted by the hospital community and its perspective. Social science research has amply demonstrated that a single person is hard pressed to maintain his or her own perspective in the face of social pressure. There is safety (and comfort) for the lay person in numbers and, perhaps more important, there is safety for the committee. If the ethics committee wants a lay person for any particular reason (and it should), then that reason must include the lay member's nonhospital perspective. The committee would do well to ensure that the lay perspective is protected and heard. Increasing the number of lay persons would serve that purpose.

References

Aroskar, M. A. Health care professionals. In: Cranford, R. E., and Doudera, A. E., eds. *Institutional Ethics Committees and Health Care Decision Making.* Ann Arbor, MI: Health Administration Press, 1984, pp. 218-25.

National Commission for the Protection of Human Subjects of Biomedical and Behavioral Research. *The Belmont Report: Ethical Principles and Guidelines for the Protection of Human Subjects of Research.* Washington, DC: U.S. Government Printing Office, 1979.

Ruddick, W., and Finn, W. Objections to hospital philosophers. *J Med Ethics.* 1985. 11:42-6.

Chapter 7

Committee Procedures

Keeping Records

Record keeping is of particular concern to ethics committees in three primary areas: the minutes of the meetings, the notes on patients' charts, and the records of committee consultations. A fourth area, which requires little discussion, includes records of the committee's work, such as guidelines and other written materials that are disseminated in the hospital as a result of committee initiative. Much of the discussion about ethics committees and record keeping has focused on fear of liability and on concerns that records not be legally discoverable. These concerns seem ill-focused for several reasons. First, because ethics committees have been created for the most part to protect patients' interests and to provide accountability to the public with respect to very controversial and difficult ethical decisions, the records ought not to be buried. Indeed, to the extent that committee records do not breach patient confidentiality, they ought to be available as a record of the committee's work. Second, because the justifications for providing strict protection of medical committee records do not clearly apply to ethics committees, it is very possible that the records may not have the same legal protection.

Patients' medical records are usually available to courts, at least in those instances in which the patient consents to their release, in which the patient has placed his medical condition at issue through litigation, or in other specifically defined instances. Because it is very possible that all relevant committee records would be available to the courts in the event of a lawsuit, the committee should assume that such would be the case and keep its records accordingly. Committees would be advised to keep good, accurate records. Should they be needed in a legal case, no one will benefit by ambiguous or inaccurate records, whether minutes of meetings, case consultation records, or other committee records.

Minutes should accurately report the committee's agenda items in policy writing, education, and case review. They should state the options available to the committee, the actions taken, and, when appropriate, the reasons that the committee chose a specific course. Minutes need not and should not be excessively detailed, but they should make clear the issues the committee considered, the conclusions they reached, and the reasons for those conclusions. If a committee develops good meeting agendas and sticks to the agendas, the minutes should flow easily from the agenda, for the minutes are an account of the progress on the agenda items. The minutes should also provide those who were unable to attend the meeting an adequate account of what transpired. The minutes should be distributed according to customary hospital policies, which vary from hospital to hospital.

A committee may want to include summaries of case reviews in the minutes or it may prefer to develop separate case review records, noting in the minutes only that a case review was conducted. Case review summary sheets might be appropriate if the committee wants to be able to quickly review its work in this area, if it intends to conduct any kind of evaluation of the case review function that would necessitate access to charts, or if the summary sheets are needed for educational purposes. However the case review records are handled, the records should not include patient names. It is inevitable that a description of the patient's situation (which would be necessary) might make it possible for someone to identify the patient. Identifying numbers should be included only if the committee knows why it needs to have that kind of identification. Some may wish to use coded numbers that would permit those with access to the code to identify patients. However, before such a coding arrangement is used, the committee would be well-advised to consider why it would want to be able to identify patients and to be sure that the benefits are very significant. Because the committee may be discussing a case without the patient's knowledge or consent, *any* risk of harm to the patient would need significant justification. (Discussing patients without their consent is examined further in relation to case review in chapter 8 and in the context of Privacy, Confidentiality, and Privilege, chapter 11.)

A committee needs to consider whether case review records should include the name of the person who brought the case to the committee's attention, the name of the attending physician, or the names of any other health care professionals who were involved in the case. Some writers have suggested that these records should provide very little specific information about those directly involved in the case and a great deal of information about the committee's advice and recommendations and the reasons for that advice. If separate consultation forms are used, they should include at a minimum the names of all those present at the committee review (committee members as well as others), a description of the clinical situation, the alternatives discussed by the committee, the committee's final advice or recommendations, and the rationale for that advice. Sample consultation forms are included in appendix C.

Writing notes on a patient's chart about ethics committee reviews is controversial. Some have suggested that the attending physician note only that an ethics conference or consultation was conducted. Others, however, have argued that if any chart note is made, it should accurately and fully describe the results of that conference. Some have suggested that the ethics committee chairman, rather than the attending physician, should write the note. Others have very strongly asserted that no mention of ethics committee consultations should ever be included in the patient's chart. There is something to be said both for and against this practice and each committee will need to assess its own situation.

Two principles might be used to guide this decision: (1) Will documenting ethics committee involvement serve to protect and further the patient's interests? (2) Will documenting ethics committee involvement increase public accountability for decisions? Clearly, making chart notes is problematic for physicians, nurses, ethics committees, and hospitals in some instances (additionally so when the patient is not aware that his or her situation has been discussed by the ethics committee and the patient has a

right to see the records). However, institutional or professional risks ought not to be the primary rationale for this decision. If a committee does decide to make chart notes, then this practice should be consistent. That is, the committee should write notes in all cases that it reviews. Although there is no consensus on the overall question of chart notes, it is our belief that if the committee is offering case review, it ought to be prepared to document its recommendations in the progress notes or on a consultation form, if hospitals choose to use consult forms for that purpose. Practices with respect to writing notes in the chart will, of course, need to conform to hospital policies.

Over time, ethics committees may find that they have generated a considerable number of documents related to the workings of the committee. Most hospitals have no single, natural home for these documents, which might range from guidelines and policies to patient brochures including information about various living wills and other patient directives. Some committees have attempted to ensure that all ethics committee documents are kept in a single notebook on each unit so that they can be easily located. Others provide documents or forms on request. Solutions to this problem should be worked out by each hospital, but committees should at least consciously address the issue of whether the educational and policy materials that they generate or introduce are in fact accessible to physicians, hospital staff, patients, and patients' families.

Subcommittees

A large committee frequently makes extensive use of subcommittees of three or four persons to carry out much of the committee's work. It is clear that an ethics committee charged with providing education, policy recommendations, and prospective or retrospective case reviews cannot achieve much in a single monthly meeting of one to two hours (the meeting time for most ethics committees). The committee may want to create either permanent or ad hoc subcommittees to carry out most of their work. Thus, for example, when the committee has decided that a new policy/guideline should be written, the actual writing and subsequent revision of the policy should be done by a subcommittee. The whole committee should avoid using meeting times to make such changes as word-by-word language revisions of the policy. Instead, committee time should be used to make conceptual revisions. Members can also suggest wording or other revisions by giving them in writing to the subcommittee. The subcommittee can then resubmit to the whole committee.

Similarly, case reviews can be conducted by subcommittees. When time is of the essence, it will be impossible to convene the entire committee. When time is available, however, it is preferable for the whole committee to provide review. Each committee needs to decide how to arrange for these rapid subcommittee reviews. It may be that specific members are designated as the review subcommittee for a specific period of time and they are on call for that purpose. Or, it may be that the committee chairman takes the responsibility for gathering together a subcommittee each time a need for prompt review arises. Whatever system is used, it is important that it be considered and understood by the whole committee. If a clear system is not constructed, then impromptu decisions about how to handle time-pressured case reviews will be necessary, and these decisions may not meet with the committee's favor. Because the subcommittee members are acting on behalf of the entire committee, it behooves the entire committee to decide how those actions are to be structured.

Much of the committee's education work also can be handled by subcommittees. The committee as a whole can give the subcommittee general guidance regarding ethics rounds, committee self-education meetings, or other activities, and the subcommittee can then be depended upon to make decisions and recommendations.

Like most committees, ethics committees tend to become bogged down in details. Thus, when 15 to 20 individuals make the effort to meet, they should ensure that the meeting time is spent in worthwhile actions. Using subcommittees to carry out all the detailed work of the committee will make it possible to use meeting times for those issues that demand the attention and the contributions of everyone.

Voting: Making Committee Decisions

Committees need to consider how to handle methods of decision making because, although they are not deciding how particular cases are handled, they must make decisions about other matters. Some committees use written ballots; some use voice votes; some use no voting at all, but permit the chairman to determine when consensus is reached. Each method has its advantages and disadvantages.

Voting as a means of decision making is appealing in a democratic society, but the committee needs to consider whether or not that is what is needed. Majority rule is not usually what is sought in an ethics committee. In case review, the committee's purpose should be to clarify the options; it is not clear how

voting can further that goal. However, requiring an individual to vote means that he or she must take a definite position. Allowing consensus decisions frequently means that more dominant individuals can control committee actions. Voice voting may be somewhat more successful than consensus determinations in achieving full participation.

If voting is used, the way it is handled may depend upon the dynamics of the individual committee. A group with problems of hierarchy or dominance among its members may want to use written ballots. A group with good rapport may find consensus determinations more efficient and perfectly adequate. Voting should not usually be conducted casually. To call for a voice vote as a "mere formality" may be adequate for minor matters, but on issues that involve substantive decisions (for example, approving a final version of a proposed policy or determining substantial committee activities), the chairman should make sure that each person is committed to a position or has specifically chosen to abstain from voting.

Group Leadership

Once the committee has passed the stage in which the primary function is self-education, meetings should be conducted in a skilled manner. Leading groups through analyses of difficult problems, arriving at sound solutions, and exploring future issues is a complex task, especially when members of the group do not normally work together. Some people come by leadership skills naturally, but most of us learn through experience—often negative experiences that teach us primarily what we do not want to do. Each group and each chairman needs to be sensitive to the problems of group dynamics. In order to help the ethics committee work as a group, we have assembled some practical suggestions from our own experience and from a training system entitled *Group Action,* designed by Zenger Miller. This information is contained in appendix D.

Committee Evaluation

Formal evaluations should be conducted at least once a year and should include self-evaluation by individual members and also evaluation of committee work as a whole. Self-evaluations should solicit the committee members' perceptions of both their own and the committee's effectiveness with respect to the members' expectations. Individual evaluations should provide for anonymity and should be conducted systematically through the use of evaluation forms that allow open-ended as well as yes/no answers. When members leave the committee, they should also be asked to provide departing evaluations unless anonymity cannot be ensured. (Additional tips on creating evaluation forms, as well as sample questions, are provided in appendix E.)

The committee chairman can also conduct informal evaluations of the members' attitudes by taking note of member attendance. Whether members attend meetings provides important information about their assessment of the committee's value. Meeting times can be a problem, but the fact is that, in the hospital, any time can be inopportune. If the members believe the work is important, they will arrange to get there, even if they must come late or leave early. Even if members are attending, the chairman may sense that something is not working well and can privately inquire of other members if they, too, sense problems and what they think those problems might be. People are often willing to say in private what they will not say in public. A good group leader can use the sensitivity of others as an extension of his or her own awareness in order to improve the effectiveness of the committee.

Formal evaluation of the committee's work involves a considerable effort, but it is essential if the committee is to serve the hospital community effectively. Usually, after an ethics committee writes or revises a policy, it also conducts some in-service training for the staff members who will be implementing the policy. Other education modes within the hospital will also be used. The committee may work with the administration to make sure that the written policy is available to everyone as well as to be certain that everyone understands it. Unfortunately, the committee then usually walks away, assuming that its work is done. If policies and guidelines are handled this way, many ethics committee members may think that formulating them is not a very worthwhile activity. Policies and guidelines are created with great effort; then they are sent away, never to be heard of again. However, if committees were to evaluate the effect of new policies regularly, they would have a better sense of the effects of their work and a better understanding of how to improve policy implementation. For example, for many years bioethics writers deplored the absence of do-not-resuscitate (DNR) policies in hospitals. As a result of this concern, many hospitals now have specific DNR policies. Some research, however, suggests that the policies are very selectively applied. DNR orders may now be charted more frequently than before the policies were written, but consideration of the wishes of the patient and family, or their knowledge about the order, may not be common, despite the fact that policies usually include something about the need for discussion with the patient or family.

Evaluating the effect of policy implementation can be fairly complex or fairly simple. Initially, it might be adequate to have ethics committee members inquire of their colleagues whether they think the policy is being followed. If there is any indication that it is not, then it may be advisable to move to a more formal level of evaluation. This can involve chart reviews, patient or staff interviews, or even hospital-wide questionnaires. (Constructing and analyzing questionnaires involves a fair degree of skill and generally should be undertaken only if the questionnaires are brief, unless the ethics committee has the help of someone with the necessary expertise.)

Education activities should also include participant evaluation. It is not necessary perhaps to prepare a formal evaluation sheet for every in-service training session, but it might be worthwhile, for example, to provide postcards (returnable by hospital mail) to give participants an opportunity to ask further questions or to make suggestions about the session. If persons do take the time to ask questions, it is vital that someone from the committee respond promptly. Most people in the hospital are happy to have a resource that can help them when they are uncertain, but that resource, if not reliably available, will quickly lose credibility.

Evaluating consultations is more difficult. The committee might want to develop a brief form that is routinely sent to any hospital staff member or physician who brings a case to the committee or who appears before the committee, focusing on whether or not the committee's involvement was helpful and, perhaps, inquiring about the final outcome of the case if it is not already known to the committee. Information may be more accurate when evaluations are anonymous but, in the case of case reviews, it may be difficult to establish anonymity. Furthermore, the committee would find it useful to be able to tie peoples' reactions to individual cases in order to gain a better sense of what the committee had done well or poorly. If a committee chooses to do case review evaluations that are not anonymous, the evaluation forms should explain why respondents are being asked to identify themselves. Evaluation of case reviews can also be conducted informally.

Even if formal evaluations of consultations are not sought from persons outside the committee, the committee itself should regularly take some time to assess the activity. Are the members comfortable with their contributions to these cases? Are the number of consultation requests increasing, falling off, or remaining constant? If the committee seeks consensus in consultation situations, does everyone understand what is meant by consensus and does everyone believe that consensus is actually being achieved? Has the committee developed consultation forms so that they can assess their role in consultations over a period of time? Do members feel that their ability to provide effective consultations has improved over time? If consultations are usually delegated to a subcommittee, do the same people always do them? Does the entire committee know about and agree with what is done on subcommittee consultations? There are many questions that can be asked about consultation, depending upon how the specific committee conducts the review function.

Evaluation means that the committee may be found wanting or may receive criticism. Frequently, that possibility, along with the sometimes cumbersome paperwork, keeps committees from conducting any type of evaluation. All committees and all people on committees can lose their independent viewpoints about what they are doing. By inviting criticism (and approval), committees can reconsider their approaches and their attitudes and can do better work. It may mean change, and nothing seems to be resisted more than change. Yet change can lead to improved personal satisfaction when we perceive that we are achieving our goals more effectively.

Chapter 8

Functions of Ethics Committees

The work of ethics committees lies in three areas. The first area is education and includes education of the committee itself, the hospital community, and the general public outside the hospital. The second area is policy and guideline recommendations. The third area is case review, both prospective and retrospective.

Education

Educating the Committee

Each committee should have an orientation session when the committee first begins functioning and again each time new members are brought onto the committee. For the sake of efficiency, it is desirable to bring groups of new members on at a single time so that the orientation can be provided for them as a group, rather than individually.

Orientation is a difficult problem because bioethics is a very large field and members are expected (or expect themselves) to learn too much too fast. Furthermore, most ethics committees are trying to do too much at this time. The issues that have brought ethics committees into being are not simply the problems of hospitals or of health care professionals. They are questions that are basic to social values. Thus, ethics committees are not the last, but the first word in this area, a fact that ethics committee members need to realize. The desirability of having lay members on the committee is one aspect of this broader context of the field. Indeed, it is possible that we will soon see mixed professional-citizen groups, both inside and outside of government, addressing these questions.

Ethics committee members will need time to develop involvement with the subject. They may need to think about what qualifies them to be a member of an ethics committee. A tendency to think that all health care professionals are already qualified, merely by virtue of their professional training, is common. Qualification, however, is more a matter of being willing to learn something new, rather than of having prior knowledge. Ethics committee members need to take their self-education seriously and be willing to spend some time and energy in learning about ethics, law, and the history of bioethics.

The committee should think of group orientation, individual self-education, and committee self-education as separate functions, although for a brand new committee the distinctions may be less obvious. Orientation for new members should include one or more sessions introducing them to bioethics, ethical decision making in health care, current important topics, and the committee's functions and goals. Orientation sessions usually take about three hours and may be split into two parts. New members should be given written materials prior to the orientation and should be expected to read them so that they are able to participate actively in the orientation session.

The first goal of orientation is to provide new members with a context for the issues that are the concern of the committee. New members need to understand what constitutes the field of bioethics and what is meant by ethical decision making in health care settings. Orientation should include a discussion of definitions and ethical distinctions. It should not be assumed that members will have a common understanding of ethics or of what constitutes an ethical issue. Committee members will need help in recognizing and sorting out key ethical principles and may need help in understanding the difference between logical argumentation and rhetorical arguments or slogans. This manual can provide much of the basic information on ethics that new ethics committee members will need. (See especially part I, "Ethics and Health Care.") The second goal of orientation is to give the new members information about the committee's previous work (if the group has been in existence for some time) and its current goals. Orientation leaders should ensure that new members understand what the committee does and does not do.

Individual self-education, which new members should pursue fairly aggressively in the first few months, includes reading relevant books and journals. This manual contains a considerable amount of material that will be helpful to new members, including an extensive bibliography. Individual self-education might also include taking a course in bioethics, perhaps one taught at a nearby community college or university extension. New members should be encouraged to attend such a class and, if the committee has sufficient funds, it might consider paying for books or tuition for the classes. In addition, many conferences on issues in bioethics are held throughout the United States and members should be encouraged to attend them, and helped to do so if possible. Usually, bioethics conferences carry continuing education credit.

Committee self-education usually focuses on discussions of books (The President's Commission's *Deciding to Forego Life-Sustaining Treatment* and Jonsen, Siegler, and Winslade's *Clinical Ethics* are very effective for this purpose), of case studies, or of audiovisual materials. Some committees devote a portion of every meeting to case studies in order to develop the committee members' facility in asking the right questions, sorting out the significant principles involved, and suggesting appropriate options. (Appendix F, "Case Studies and Analyses," provides sample case studies for this purpose.) Many committees have occasional consultants from outside the hospital who either make presentations to the committee on specific topics (for example, the principles of ethical analysis, the legal status of patient directives, and so forth) or facilitate committee discussions, helping the members to consider different perspectives. Staff and physicians from within the hospital should also be considered as important resources in ensuring that all members of the committee possess the necessary medical, nursing, and social work information—such information as brain death determination; artificial feeding techniques; adoption, foster care, or other placement for disabled children; side effects of dialysis treatment; and relevance of the various professional

codes of ethics. It is important to remember that, despite the fact that most ethics committee members work in the hospital, they do not necessarily share a common body of information about medical care. Committees are interdisciplinary just so that the members can learn from one another. Part of committee self-education should address that learning in a formal way.

For many committees, questions about terminating treatment will be a central focus. Members should be familiar with both the medical and the legal aspects of this issue. They should know case law, both in their own state and in other states (see chapter 14, "Landmark Cases"). Committee members should know about their own state's legislation on the definition of death, living wills, durable powers of attorney, and natural death acts. They should be cognizant of the differences between the various patient directives. Withholding CPR and writing do-not-resuscitate orders pose a number of potential problems and members should be aware of the discussions of this issue, as well as the guidelines that local medical and bar associations may have suggested for withholding treatment.

Committee self-education should include opportunities not only for learning about ethics and ethical principles but also for applying that learning to hypothetical or actual (retrospective) cases. It should formally address legal concepts and important legal cases (see part III). In addition to these substantive areas, some committees take a few sessions specifically to discuss their own basic attitudes, values, and feelings about bioethics issues. This can be difficult to do, and may require an outside leader, but when successful is extremely effective in enhancing group functioning by expanding the members' senses of knowing and understanding one another.

Educating the Hospital Community

After the committee has embarked on the process of self-education, it may also want to begin education for the entire hospital community. The committee members need not feel that they themselves must supply the education for the hospital community. Especially at the beginning, this may require outside speakers or hospital staff or physicians with specialized knowledge. Thus, educating the hospital community can proceed simultaneously with the committee members' own education.

Two customary forms of hospital education used by many ethics committees are ethics rounds and ethics conferences. Ethics rounds are intended to attract a smaller audience (frequently, members of a department or unit), whereas ethics conferences are usually addressed to the entire hospital community. Ethics rounds usually address a single case, either actual or hypothetical, and give participants a chance to see how ethical problems can be dealt with. Topics for ethics conferences, which are likely to be longer than ethics rounds, might include discussions and formal presentations on *Deciding to Forego Life-Saving Treatment;* on new laws, such as the durable power of attorney; on case discussions of highly publicized cases (for example, the *Elizabeth Bouvia* case); or on a discussion of current issues (for example, withholding food and fluids).

When providing education for the hospital community, the ethics committee must be clear about its target audience, whether it be the entire hospital community, patients and families, the nursing units, the ancillary professions, the medical staff, or the administrative staff. Sometimes, educational programs can be provided that will attract all these groups. For the most part, however, each committee will have to decide who it can or needs to reach, and then develop education programs appropriately. Timing, subjects, and follow-up all would be affected by audience choice.

The development of new policies or guidelines is an important mode of hospital community education. Some committees use the in-service training associated with newly approved policies as an educational opportunity. Other committees use draft policies as the focus of staff and physician discussions. One ethics committee sponsored an open meeting to discuss its DNR policy draft. The session was multidisciplinary and the ensuing dialogue extremely enlightening and long overdue. As a result, the guidelines were significantly revised and another general meeting planned. Using drafts creates an opportunity both to stimulate thinking and to develop among the staff some sense of general involvement in policy development. This may be especially important if the committee thinks there may be some resistance to new policies.

Some ethics committees use commercially prepared videotapes for education, arranging to show them on the unit, followed by a discussion led by an ethics committee member. The video equipment is then left on the unit for a day or two so that the film can also be seen by those who were unable to see it the first time. The ethics committee member who led the discussion should be available for further questions, if only by telephone.

One of the most important considerations in providing effective education is whether there is any possibility of follow-up. Frequently, participants have questions only later, either when they have had time to consider the issue or when the issue arises in a practical context. No single education presentation can answer all the questions an audience member might ever have, but if people know that they can later go to someone if they do have questions, then the committee is providing ongoing assistance and the possibility of ongoing education. Whenever the committee conducts or sponsors an educational activity, it should make sure that the members of the audience know that they can come back to the committee for further information later, should it be needed. Of course, the committee cannot be expected to provide everything, but it should be able to help the individual to find information and to understand the issue better.

Some hospital employees who are involved in patient care are often overlooked with respect to bioethics education. This may include dietitians, respiratory therapists, and pharmacists. In addition, employees who are not directly involved in patient care, such as clerical workers and housekeepers, are also interested in these issues. Some committees have conducted regular "brown bag" luncheon discussions for these groups. If the committee members expect to conduct education programs themselves and are uncertain of their skills, they may want to start with this group. Such hospital workers are usually very interested in and enthusiastic about these topics. The fact that they represent a "lay" audience may be helpful when the committee begins education programs for the lay community outside the hospital.

Some committees have reported doing staff surveys to determine the staff's greatest concerns. Subsequently, the committees focused their educational efforts in these areas. One hospital surveyed their physicians on attitudes and behaviors regarding informed consent and found several areas in need of discussion and policy making. In another hospital, a physician survey showed that many physicians were interested in learning more about ethics topics that were not directly within their speciality work. Thus, for example, interest in information about treatment of seriously ill newborns was expressed by physicians throughout the hospital.

Ethics committees frequently ask how they can ensure physician attendance at educational programs. This appears to be a problem at many hospitals. Probably the most effective way to deal with this is to target some programs specifically for medical staff and integrate them into the existing continuing medical education conducted by the medical education department. If the director of the education department is particularly interested in ethics issues, he or she can help in providing occasional forums for ethics education at medical staff or medical education meetings.

When seeking to involve physicians in broader audience programs, it may help to involve some of them as presenters. Using actual cases from the hospital will involve some as participant-presenters. Other physicians with special expertise might be invited to participate as discussants or as resources. For example, at one hospital, an ethics conference on brain death included a member of the medical staff who had been involved in the Harvard ad hoc committee. Similarly, a staff neurologist might be included to explain the technical aspects of brain death determination.

Educating the Lay Community

The lay community is very interested in bioethical issues. By targeting the general public for educational activities, the ethics committee can reach future patients. This group is probably most interested in how to control one's own decisions in health care. Therefore, any kind of education about patient directives (durable powers of attorney, natural death acts, living wills, uniform anatomical gift acts) or do-not-resuscitate orders is likely to be well received. Evening or weekend programs are most likely to attract community audiences. These can be held at the hospital, but may be more successful in a more neutral setting. Some towns have community meetings or town hall forums. If so, the ethics committee may want to propose that a forum be conducted on ethical issues in health care.

Lay audiences are also interested in learning more about how to talk to their doctor in order to ensure that they know what is happening and how to participate in decision making. In addition, they are interested in such issues as how and when to call ambulances, an area of discussion involving patients' wishes to receive the maximum treatment that is available. This is especially important in connection with patient directives. People who do not want to have all possible treatment are often unclear about the relationship between calling for emergency care and asserting patient desires to refuse treatment. Thus, a program about the ethical dimensions of providing emergency care would be appropriate and useful. In general, the nonhospital community needs the same education as does the ethics committee itself, although the education that can be provided in a single session for the general audience is likely to be less complex.

Writing Policies and Guidelines

Because thoughtful and carefully written policies can have a substantial effect on health care decisions, it is particularly important that ethics committee members take the writing of policies very seriously. Writing good policies is often a slow, time-consuming process that can prove very frustrating to health care professionals who are oriented to faster and more concrete results. In the past, committees have been more likely to recommend *guidelines,* which are only advisory, rather than *policies,* which are mandatory, primarily because they were not always certain of their authority or mandate.

It is our belief that the committee should recommend policies rather than guidelines whenever the committee has reached consensus regarding a standard of ethical practice. For example, if there is general consensus that a DNR order should not be written for a competent patient unless he or she consents to the order's being written, the issue should be addressed in a policy, not in a guideline. In areas where there is uncertainty or disagreement about the appropriate way to approach an ethical issue, guidelines are appropriate. As attitudes evolve, however, it may be necessary to change guidelines to policies to ensure standard ethical practices.

If there are general expectations about what practices are appropriate, it is misleading to characterize those expectations as guidelines, implying that individuals may choose to follow them or not, as their own thoughts suggest. Although policies are mandatory, it should be understood that a given policy may still allow for discretionary judgments in specific instances or in specific areas of the policy.

Following are some considerations that the committee can use in developing policies. It is assumed that, before an ethics committee begins to make policy recommendations, its governing body (medical executive committee, administration, or governing board) has authorized that as an appropriate function.

Policies should be as brief as possible (for ease of reference) without sacrificing important content. Some committees have found that the policies they write are necessarily lengthy but that an abbreviated version can be prepared for ordinary use.

A policy has four elements: a statement of the policy, a statement of principles, a list of definitions, and a list of procedures.

Statement of the Policy

This is a brief statement that summarizes the general topic of the policy, giving the general case and its major exceptions. It may also add to the general case.

The following are examples of policy statements:

- Newborn infants must receive life-saving treatment unless treatment would be futile or would prolong their dying. All infants, regardless of prognosis, must receive appropriate food and fluids and standard nursing care.

- Patients who suffer cardiac or pulmonary arrest must receive cardiopulmonary resuscitation (CPR) unless a do-not-resuscitate (DNR) order has been written in the patient's chart.
- All permanently unconscious patients must receive food and hydration adequate to sustain their lives unless the family or other legally authorized individual gives specific written consent to withhold food or fluids.

Statement of Principles

This is a listing of the relevant principles and values that underlie the policy. These statements are implicitly or specifically prefaced by the statement "We believe that. . . ." The statement of principles may, at hospitals sponsored by religious groups, include specifically theological principles. At secular hospitals, the principles are more likely to be articulated in terms of philosophical discourse. The principles, however, need not use specifically philosophical language. Ethical principles may be expressed in ordinary language and continue to remain statements of belief. Note that the principles are not about facts, for example, they are not statements about legal realities such as: "Informed consent is required before treating a patient in a nonemergency situation" or "A patient who meets brain-death criteria is dead." These are factual statements that are either true or false because, as a matter of fact, informed consent is required and because criteria for death are legally defined in the United States.

Principles should be included so that ethics committee members, members of the hospital community (including patients), and the general public can understand what values the hospital is espousing for these value-laden decisions. It also ensures that there is an ethical basis for the policies. Many people make value judgments intuitively, but a specific articulation of the principles ensures that the ethical concerns have been clearly thought out and the ethical dilemma resolved in a specific manner.

The following are examples of statements of principles:

- Because life is valued, life-saving treatment should always be provided in cases of uncertainty (sanctity of life).
- Competent patients may refuse life-saving treatment as long as they fully understand the implications of

their choice and the possibilities of any other treatment (autonomy).

- Information about patients and their families should not be revealed to persons who are not involved in the patient's care without the patient's consent or a legal requirement (confidentiality).
- Because competent patients have the legal and moral right to make their own choices, health care providers must always give accurate and adequate information (truth telling).
- Health care professionals should not be required to act in opposition to their consciences (autonomy).
- When life-sustaining treatment is foregone, health care professionals have an obligation to provide maximum care and comfort to the patient (beneficence).

List of Definitions

All ambiguous terms in the policy must be clearly defined so that interpretation of the policy does not lead to substantially varying, unintended results. Clear definitions will ensure that policies can be reliably interpreted by different people at different times. Although the definition section is the third element of the policy, it may need to be written last. That is, after completing several drafts of the policy, the ethics committee needs to go through the text and determine which words or phrases need to be defined. In this process, omissions or logical lapses in the policy often become apparent. Often the terms to be defined do not have exact meanings. As a result, each hospital may define them in slightly different ways. This is perfectly acceptable. For example, hospital A may decide that *imminent* means within a week, whereas hospital B may use it to mean during the current hospitalization. Either definition is acceptable because it is *specific for that hospital*. That is, it makes clear how people at that hospital are to interpret the word.

Some commonly undefined and ambiguous words include:

- Terminal or terminal illness.
- Imminent death.
- Consult (for example, The physician must consult with the incompetent patient's family). Does this mean to inform them of the decision that the physician has already made, to ask them what decision they wish to make, to ask them to consent to the decision made by the physician, or merely to make sure they do not oppose the decision? The use of the word consult makes it unclear where the decision-making authority lies.

- Competent/incompetent patient. Although competency is a legal term, in policies it does not usually refer to a legal judgment. Policies seldom define what it means or who determines the state.
- Proportionate/disproportionate treatment. These phrases are much preferred to such older terms as ordinary, extraordinary, or heroic treatment. Whatever terms are used to characterize the degree of treatment should be defined. The words proportionate and disproportionate, for example, involve a judgment about the burdens of treatment or nontreatment. Whose perspective is to be considered when making that judgment?
- Quality of life. This term, if used, must be carefully defined, especially with respect to how quality is to be measured and from whose perspective.
- Medical procedures. Such terms as cardiopulmonary rescuscitation (CPR) and do-not-resuscitate (DNR) orders may need to be defined in order to make clear what they mean in a particular hospital.

List of Procedures

Procedures are the specific, pragmatic steps that are to be taken in order to implement the policy. Procedures include such matters as what is to be recorded in the chart, who is to be consulted in the event of disagreements, and who is to be informed in the event of certain actions. Thus, the procedures for treating seriously ill newborns might include such statements as, "Before recommending that life-prolonging treatment be withdrawn, consult those within the hospital who have special expertise in the infant's disorder." Or, "If physicians and nurses disagree about an adult patient's competency to refuse treatment, contact the hospital ethics committee." Procedures should include instructions on what to do when there is disagreement among the relevant decision makers. If the statement is only advisory, the word *may* is to be used with the verb. If the statement is mandatory, then *must* or *will* is appropriate. Thus, *physicians may* or *physicians will or must* do this or provide that. It is advisable to avoid *shall* or *should* when writing procedures because there may be confusion as to whether *should* implies an obligation or is simply conditional. Thus, for example, "Doctors should document the DNR order in the medical record" may mean that he or she must do so or it may mean that he or she should do so, but that there may be reasons for not doing so in some cases. At best, the word *should* implies a general principle rather than a rule or specific procedure. To avoid confusion, avoid using it in the procedures section.

The following are examples of written procedures:

- Physicians will write the DNR order in the medical record and also include, in the progress notes, a justification for that order.
- When the parents of an infant with a life-threatening condition refuse treatment for the infant, consult the ethics committee.
- Before writing a DNR order for an incompetent patient with no family or legal surrogate, request a second opinion from another physician who has not previously been involved in the patient's care.
- If care givers disagree about a patient's competency, seek a consultation from a psychiatrist or request a legal ruling.
- If the care givers believe that treatment is morally and perhaps legally required, but the family disagrees, the primary physician must consult either the ethics committee or the risk management committee.
- Surrogate decision makers are to use the *substituted judgment* standard for decisions relating to incompetent patients rather than the *best interests* standards, whenever possible.

Drafting Policies

First, determine which topics or issues need to be the subjects of policies. (Examples include, but are not limited to, administrative procedures for stopping treatment for patients who meet brain-death criteria, do-not-resuscitate orders, foregoing treatment and supportive care orders, criteria for patients in ICUs, treatment of seriously ill newborns, the use of patient preference documents, and good decision making practices.) This decision should not be arbitrary. Rather, the committee should be aware of specific problems that would be helped by the existence of policies. Furthermore, the issue should occur with some frequency. On one hand, if only one or two problem cases arise in a particular area, then the problem may not require a policy. On the other hand, although problems with patients meeting brain-death criteria arise infrequently, a policy is very helpful in such cases.

Second, gather pertinent information and sample policies used by other hospitals, or similar policies from within the hospital, and appraise them critically. Some sample policies are included in *Deciding to Forego Life-Sustaining Treatment* (the President's Commission) and *Institutional Ethics Committees and Health Care Decision Making* (Cranford and Doudera). Do not—at least without careful consideration—simply adopt another hospital's policy. Some writers have suggested that it is unnecessary for each ethics committee to invent the wheel and that it

is more efficient if the committee uses already existing policies and simply adapts them to meet their own
needs.[1] It is our opinion, however, that much can be
learned from writing policies and that many important issues are lost if the committee does not carefully
consider what is to go into its own policy. Although
there is no need for everyone to reinvent the wheel,
it behooves everyone to understand how the parts of
the wheel work. Certainly, the committee should look
at policies used by other hospitals. When using examples from other committees, members should be concerned with comparing their differences and assessing
the meaning of those differences.

Third, when writing policies, make sure that it is
clear whether actions or decisions are mandatory or
discretionary. The language chosen can easily obscure
this distinction and it is vital for those who are
implementing the policies to know what they must do
and what they may do, what is required and what is
discretionary. Thus, for example, the use of the word
should can lead to considerable uncertainty about
meaning. *Should* implies obligation, but it is also a
conditional form. In a statement of principle, *should*
is appropriately used because the intention is to make
a general statement, not a rule. A principle differs
from a rule in that a principle provides guidance
whereas a rule gives directions. Consider the difference between *People should not steal* and *People will
not steal (or must not steal)*. The latter is much
stronger with respect to determining conduct.

Thus, *should* may be appropriately used in stating principles but not in stating procedures. If the
action in the procedure is discretionary, the appropriate language is *may* or *might*. If it is obligatory, then
will or *must* should be used. There can be a problem
with trying to make policies too precise, but that is
probably less of a problem than making them too
vague with ambiguous language.

Fourth, closely assess the language in all segments
of the policy. Evaluate it for clarity and practical
application. Is it filled with technical language or jar-
gon? Make sure that the language can be understood.
Avoid the use of the passive voice as much as possible (for example, "X may be done"). The passive voice
focuses on what is to be done, but not on who is to
do it. Usually, those who must follow policies need
to know who is supposed to do what, not just what
is to be done. Test out the policy on a few persons
who were not in on the committee's discussion to see
if any areas are ambiguous, unclear, or open to abuse.
Similarly, if policies are to be available to patients and
their families, the language level must be carefully
assessed. Health care professionals often do not realize how much technical language they use and how

inscrutable it is to patients. Writing in simple English
is difficult but essential if the policies are to be useful
to patients. In addition, when the policies are to be
available to patients, they should be available in trans-
lation if a significant number of patients speak a
different language as their primary tongue.

Fifth, if there are internal sanctions, state them
in the policy. Although administrative policies usually
do not include legal sanctions, there is a risk of liability when hospital policies are not followed. The
medical executive committee may wish to support policies recommended by the ethics committee with internal sanctions, as well.

Sixth, when the committee has completed several
drafts (rewriting is mandatory), consult knowledgeable staff members (who may not be on the committee) to be sure that the policy addresses practical
concerns in an appropriate way.

Seventh, before the policy is accepted by the institution, have it reviewed by legal counsel if that is
hospital practice. Do not try to anticipate the objections that lawyers might make. If they have concerns,
they will make them known in time, but the committee need not inhibit its own best thoughts and judgments by fears about legal issues. Of course, the
committee will not make recommendations that they
know to be illegal. Our concern here is that the committee not restrict its own best thinking by worrying
about the objections of hospital lawyers looking for
liability issues.

Finally, develop a process whereby the committee can obtain feedback and comments from hospital
staff while the policies are still in draft form. This
serves several purposes: first, it helps to educate those
who review the documents about the subtle issues;
second, it provides additional information that will
strengthen the completed document; and third, the
policy is more likely to be accepted if those outside
the committee have had an opportunity to contribute
and to have their concerns addressed. The process of
obtaining feedback from the staff should continue
even after the policy is put into effect so that any mis-
understanding on the part of the staff members acting on the policy can be resolved.

Implementation

To implement the policies it has written, the ethics
committee should clarify the lines of authority and
responsibility for approving and revising policies. Who
must approve them? Who will distribute them? Who
will be responsible for answering questions that arise
about their meaning or their interpretation? The committee should develop a method for educating the

hospital community regarding the policies. It is insufficient simply to distribute them once they are approved. In addition, it should develop a method for evaluating the effectiveness of the policies and for reviewing and revising them when necessary.

Reviewing Cases

Taking On the Role of Case Reviewer

Persons who are uncertain about the value of ethics committees in hospitals are particularly wary about committees providing case review or case consultation, as it is frequently called. Their fear is that the committees will, at the very least, intrude upon the doctor-patient relationship and, at worst, either directly or indirectly take over decision-making authority. This fear is a realistic one, and committees should be very cautious about taking on a case review function. It is probably unwise for a new committee to begin its work by offering case reviews. Even after an initial period of self-education, committees would be well advised to give their attention to policy development and hospital community education.

Perhaps ethics committees tend naturally to want to take on the case review role because it is closer to the action, more immediately useful, and sometimes more rewarding than the slow process of providing education (with its very low-key rewards) or of developing policies (with its bureaucratic frustration). As well, once committees are established, they may be asked to review cases even before they are ready to do so. They can, of course, say no, as long as they are not required by either the hospital or the law to review specific cases. (No law requires committees to review cases at this time.) Nevertheless, this is one of those areas where dragons are likely to be lurking, and ethics committees are advised to proceed very slowly and cautiously.

For an ethics committee to fill a case review function effectively, the members must have the capacity to care about the opinions of fellow members, be comfortable with their understanding of ethical thinking and analysis, and have a high degree of credibility within the hospital community. Self-education, hospital-community education, and policy and guideline development will make the first two possible. Credibility, however, must be earned by good works. Some committees have sought to attain instant credibility by making sure that the ethics committee counts among its members only prestigious or authoritative physicians or high-ranking hospital staff persons. Although this will probably give the ethics commit-

tee *initial* credibility—or at least the benefit of the doubt—the committee will have to build its credibility by what its members do as a *group,* not by who they are as *individuals*. It cannot be assumed that a committee of prestigious, authoritative individuals (for example, the heads of all the services) will be able to work together effectively. That is, the whole is probably not equal to the sum of its parts: it may be more, or it may be less.

The ethics committee should use its role as educator and as policy developer to demonstrate to the hospital community why it can be trusted to provide responsible case review that does not usurp the physician's role. The committee will be more likely to achieve this trust by consistently seeking the hospital community's responses to committee work, by offering its services to all members of the community, and by remaining open about what it is doing. Submitting drafts of new policies to the hospital community for comment and offering ample opportunity to hear anyone who disagrees will help to create that credibility.

Education efforts that appeal to all segments of the hospital community, not just to a selected group, will also make a difference. For example, some ethics committees have found nurses far more responsive than physicians to educational programs. A decision, born of frustration, to focus education on nursing personnel (because they appreciate it or welcome it) will perhaps increase the committee's sense of satisfaction with its work, but it will not be sufficient to build its credibility. This is not to suggest that all education programs must appeal to everyone, but rather that no segment of the community should be ignored, even if it does not seem interested and even if the education process is frustrating for the committee.

Finally, the committee should attempt to keep the hospital community regularly apprised of what it is doing through whatever vehicles of communication the hospital has. Although the hospital "grapevine" is the fastest method of providing information, it is, unfortunately, not the most accurate. In the early stages, especially before case review has begun, committees might consider opening all or some of their meetings to anyone who cares to attend. They may want to invite one or two nonmembers to each meeting. They should seek out opportunities to provide information about their work through newsletters and should solicit the assistance of others in the hospital in presenting educational programs. It must be remembered that the members of hospital ethics committees do not have a corner on ethics. Although American culture (including hospital culture) has a particular affinity for experts and expertise, most people believe they have something important to say about ethics and morality. If credibility is to be earned and maintained, then ethics committees will have to demonstrate that they are merely taking on a formalized role with respect to ethics considerations, not the role of moral expert.

Case Review: What Is It Called?

More often than not, the case review function of the ethics committee is referred to as *consultation*. Several writers have recently questioned the validity (as well as the wisdom) of using this term.[2] In the hospital, the attending or primary physician frequently calls upon consultants or asks for consultations, and thus it is easy to see why the ethics committee's role might be referred to as that of a consultant, because it involves asking someone else for advice. The implicit nature of a medical consultation, however, is that the opinion of someone with a high level of specialized expertise is being solicited and that the specialist's advice will be followed, unless there is a very pressing reason not to do so. The members of an ethics committee are not ethical specialists or experts. They are members of a committee that is responsible for considering the ethical nature of medical decisions, and they are members of the hospital community who have a special interest in the area of ethics and have, perhaps, studied and considered ethical considerations somewhat more than their colleagues. To refer to them as consultants or to their activities as performing consultations would be to falsely represent the relationship between the committee and the health care providers and patients whom they are to serve. Furthermore, it would tend to encourage the ethics committee members to think of themselves as specialists whose opinions should be followed. In addition, consultants customarily have a direct relationship with the patient, which is not typical of an ethics committee conducting case reviews.

Despite Shakespeare's admonition, "What's in a name? That which we call a rose by any other name would smell as sweet," we know that the language we use strongly affects how we perceive the world and ourselves. Before an ethics committee begins to provide case review, the members should consider carefully exactly what service they intend to provide and what language best characterizes that service. Some committees provide a forum for discussions of troubling cases; some conduct case reviews; others structure a case conference; a Colorado committee offers explanations of various ethical options; and still others straightforwardly provide consultations. The legal and ethical consultation service of one California psy-chiatric hospital expects to determine how a case is handled with respect to legal constraints. Whenever prospective case reviews are mandatory, it may be that the opinion of the ethics committee is more like that of a standard medical consultant. The health provider who chooses not to follow that advice must be prepared to explain why he or she chose a course other than that recommended by the ethics committee: in that limited instance, the committee is an authoritative consultant.

Choosing Appropriate Issues for Case Review

If it is in the business of conducting case reviews, the ethics committee faces two distinct problems about determining what kinds of issues it is to handle. First, every ethical problem is not necessarily the business of the committee. Racial discrimination in personnel selection is an ethical (as well as legal) problem, but it is not a matter within the purview of most ethics committees. The ethics about which most ethics committees are concerned is limited to ethical problems in the clinical care of patients. Second, many problems that the committee might consider are not basically ethical problems, although they may have minor ethical components. Problems brought to the committee may be matters of faulty or nonexistent communication, or of misunderstandings about policies and guidelines. In such instances, everyone involved in clinical care may be in agreement about the important values, but working at cross-purposes. The ethics committee can be very helpful in untangling such confusion or misperceptions, but such "management" is not actually providing reviews on ethical matters.

When the hospital's governing board, medical executive committee, or chief executive officer decides that certain cases must be reviewed, the committee is likely to know the nature of the cases it will hear. However, in the absence of mandatory reviews, an ethics committee will find it very difficult—and perhaps impossible—to decide ahead of time what kinds of problems they will be willing to hear. As they respond to requests for assistance, they will understand more clearly what is possible and what is not, what is reasonable and what is not. Personnel problems, case management problems, legal problems, and communication failures are all likely to present themselves to the ethics committee in the guise of ethical problems. Some of them will turn out to be real ethical conflicts; some of them will not. The ethics committee could appropriately decide to try to give its assistance to the problems that are not intrinsically ethical, but the members should be aware of the kinds of cases they are accepting and the kinds of resolutions they are offering.

Frequently, ethical conflicts can be eliminated if the case can be managed slightly differently, if decisions can be postponed, or if injured feelings can be soothed. For example, a case that presents itself as a conflict between the patient's desire to refuse urgently needed treatment and the physician's desire to protect the patient's well-being may be resolved on a case management level by persuading the patient to wait a few days before making a decision and by persuading the physician to wait a few days before attempting to impose treatment (assuming that a few days will lead, at most, only to some worsening of the patient's condition, but not to significant or irreparable harm. The ethics committee's function might be to help the physician see other ways to manage the case so that the ethical conflict is eliminated. In such a case, the ethics committee will discuss the ethical aspects of the situation, even though the course of action taken does not involve resolving an ethical conflict.

Although ethics committees can be very helpful in matters that are not strictly ethical in character, committee members should attempt to characterize the nature of the problem before them and ask themselves: Is this really a problem that should come to us? Would another hospital committee or hospital official more appropriately handle this issue? The ethics committee cannot serve as ombudsman for the entire hospital, if for no other reason than that its members have limited time and must be available for those cases that fall uniquely within their bailiwick. Institutional review boards (IRB), quality assurance committees, utilization review committees, and risk management committees are four hospital groups whose concerns may be duplicated by the ethics committee and whose assistance should be sought if there appears to be an overlap (see "Committee Overlap," in chapter 9). For example, if a nurse brings a concern about the consent process for a therapeutic research project to the ethics committee, the committee should probably not ask that the complaint simply be refiled with the IRB. Instead, the ethics committee might want to take the matter to the attention of the IRB, in the nurse's stead, to determine whether the problem applies only to individual patients or to the informed consent protocol itself.

When and if an ethics committee decides to do case reviews, it must communicate this intention to the hospital community. It helps to establish the ethics committee's authenticity if the hospital medical director, the chief administrative officer, or the governing board (whichever is appropriate) gives the procedure its imprimatur by writing a memorandum to all concerned persons explaining the ethics committee's availability for case review. Word-of-mouth communication is probably an adequate method for getting review requests to the committee, but it is not ideal for ensuring accurate understanding or authority. The ethics committee could provide several continuing education programs for various segments of the hospital community that would serve both to announce their willingness to review cases and to explain how the procedure works. Because some health care workers may continue to be concerned about the role the ethics committee intends to play with regard to case review (they may be apprehensive of intrusion on physicians' responsibilities), an education session would be an excellent opportunity to explain exactly what the committee is and is not prepared to offer to those who bring cases to it.

In addition, if patients or their families can directly request the ethics committee to review a case, then that must be communicated in some way to patients. One ethics committee has printed a small brochure explaining the committee's functions. This brochure is routinely given to patients upon admission. It is easy to ignore the problem of informing patients because it is difficult to decide how best to do it. Most patients are probably not aware of hospital ethics committees at this time. However, over time and with continued media attention, public awareness is likely to grow and patients may ask about the availability of an ethics committee. Critics have argued that patients ought not to be routinely informed about ethics committees because they will become a focus for all their complaints. This suggests that physicians and hospital staff ought to serve as "gatekeepers" to case review because they are in a better position to understand what kind of matters the ethics committee can reasonably be expected to address. Both viewpoints have some merit, but the committee needs to consider when, if, and how patients and families are to be informed about the availability of the ethics committee, should they find themselves in an ethical conflict with their physician or the hospital staff and the physician or staff members are unwilling to consult the committee.

Prospective Review

Must Some Cases Have Mandatory Review?

As a matter of hospital policy, the ethics committee may be required to review some cases. (We urge that this not be required as an initial function of new committees.) Prior to beginning case reviews, the ethics committee should consult with the appropriate hospital authorities about what kinds of cases (if any) should be subject to mandatory review. The most commonly suggested mandatory review is that of foregoing life-sustaining treatment for an infant. The 1984 federal amendments, frequently referred to as the *Baby Doe law,* and its accompanying regulations suggest, but do not require, case review for all instances in which infants do not receive life-sustaining treatment. However, an ethics committee review might be different from the review suggested by these amendments. That is because the infant care review committees described by the regulations are not expected to make ethical assessments of treatment decisions. Instead, they are required only to determine whether or not the treatment prescribed falls within the standards of the regulations. An ethics committee, on the other hand, would be expected to address the ethical aspects of decisions in a straightforward manner. Treatment consents or refusals for adult incompetent patients who have no families are usually handled by court-appointed conservators. In the future, this could be an area for mandatory review.

Once the kinds of cases requiring mandatory review have been identified, the ethics committee should establish a method of informing the hospital community about these required reviews, including careful and specific instructions about how to submit the case for review and about the purpose and manner of the review. The committee may request that cases be submitted orally to the chairman, to any member, or to the committee secretary, or they may want more formal methods involving written requests for review. If reviews are to result in chart notes, this, too, should be publicized as part of the standard procedure.

The ability or, perhaps, the willingness of physicians and hospital staff to absorb additional bureaucratic requirements should not be overestimated. They may easily become aware of the new requirement, but remain uncertain about how to respond to it. The committee may need to prepare a new form (possibly called a mandatory review report) to be filled out and sent to the ethics committee whenever an appropriate case arises. The ethics committee may need to ensure that it has a phone that will be answered reliably by someone capable of handling the information appropriately. The committee (with administrative approval) may need to specify who has the responsibility for doing the reporting — if no one is responsible, it is likely that no one will do it. Each ethics committee will establish procedures according to its own circumstances. However, if the committee expects certain kinds of cases to come to it automatically, then it must effectively communicate both that expectation and the procedures by which the expectation can be realized. If reporting procedures are vague or difficult, then reporting will not be done and the ethics committee is likely to have little time to find these cases on its own. At least in the beginning, compliance will be voluntary; thus, it should be easy.

Who Brings Optional Case Reviews to the Committee?

Some ethics committees accept cases for review only from physicians. This may be a way to start if there is substantial physician opposition to ethics committee review of individual cases. In the long run, however, it runs counter to the philosophy behind the formation of ethics committees. It must be realized that one impetus to the formation of ethics committees was the belief of many hospital staff persons, especially nurses, that decisions were being made without sufficient consideration of ethical concerns. To restrict access to the ethics committee to physicians would certainly exacerbate those tensions even more. It might also make the ethics committee's position very difficult because its members will inevitably hear about cases involving substantial ethical problems. If they have no access to these cases other than through exerting peer pressure on their physician colleagues, then the members themselves may begin to be seen as a kind of enforcement agency. Such a result would seriously undermine not only the educational role of the ethics committee but also the prospect of developing a hospital *community* through the work of the ethics committee. The idea behind ethics committees is that all members of the hospital community, including physicians, nurses, social workers, pastoral care representatives, and administrators, should have access to the committee's services. If such a structure is not initially possible, it should be the long-term goal.

The question of providing patients with direct access to the ethics committee is also fairly controversial. Few patients even know about the committee's existence, so they are unlikely to pursue case review independently. However, insofar as the ethics committee's ultimate responsibility is to protect the patient's welfare (which includes the patient's rights), it seems logically wrong to exclude the patient or the patient's family from direct access to the committee. There is probably some tendency to want to exclude the patient from access because, despite the fact that the hospital exists to serve the patient, the patient is traditionally the "outsider" in the hospital. Patients may benefit from hospital care, but they are not members of the hospital "club." When committees decide to exclude patients from the list of those who may bring cases to the ethics committee, that exclusion may reflect a judgment of the patient and family as "outsiders" and should be reexamined.

Other, more legitimate issues might encourage committees to limit or screen patient access to the committee. Because patients and families frequently feel isolated and intimidated in hospital settings, they may seek to use the ethics committee as a hospital ombudsman. Such a role is clearly beyond the expected function of the ethics committee. (Social workers, who are trained to deal with family dynamics, may be particularly useful in assisting to resolve these patient problems.) Additionally, because patients and families may feel they have little leverage in a hospital setting, they may want to use the ethics committee to talk to their physician *for* them. This, too, will place the ethics committee in an inappropriate role that might well be destructive, both to the sense of hospital community and to the ethics committee itself, in very short order. The question of patient access to the ethics committee is a knotty one, but committees need to think seriously about how they can best help patients, without treating them as if they were troublesome children or incompetent adults. Certainly, if patients never know about the existence of a hospital ethics committee, the probability of their seeking access is small. But secrecy is the kind of solution that will inevitably backfire.

Who Sits in on Case Reviews and Who Is Informed That a Case Has Been Referred?

Assuming that the question of who can bring a case before the committee is resolved, the next questions are whether those involved in the case are informed of the referral and whether they may participate in any or all of the review procedures. Some committees discuss the case with the health care professionals who are involved in order to collect adequate information, but permit only committee members to be present during discussions. Others invite those involved to attend most of the case discussion but conduct the final discussions leading to committee recommendations with only committee members present. Others may include the physicians, the social workers, and the nurses involved in the case in all discussions. Still others hold discussions with everyone who wishes to attend; then the *committee* withdraws, leaving the final resolution to the primary care givers and the family. We believe that committees should routinely inform the physicians and all other involved caretakers when a case has been referred to the committee, inviting them to attend the case discussion.

Treating patients with respect means that patients (or their families) and the families of minors or other incompetent patients should be informed of an impending review. Determining if patients and/or family members should be present at the ethics committee review may require case-by-case decisions. In general, they should be invited to attend unless there is a specific reason not to invite them. At the very least, committee members should talk directly to them to ensure that the committee has adequate and correct information about the patient's or the family's preferences, attitudes, and values, rather than relying solely on the interpretations of others.

If case review is considered part of the process of patient care, then the patient's *permission* to conduct the review is not necessary, because he or she has already consented to sharing information among health care professionals involved in direct care. It is extremely important, however, to give *notice* to the patient whenever the ethics committee conducts a case review. It is more difficult to assess the importance of patient notice when case conferences, involving only one or two members of the ethics committee, are held spontaneously on the floor. Here, where no votes are taken or recommendations made, the nature of the "review" seems amorphous. When prior notice is difficult because of time constraints, it may suffice to inform patients afterwards that the consultation was sought. Committees should consider and be sensitive to the need to devise reasonable and ethically sensitive policies about notifying patients when ethics committee case reviews are conducted.

Some writers state categorically that patients (or their families) should always be given notice of, and even asked for consent to, an ethics committee review. However, a flat requirement of notice brings many troublesome questions. Requiring patient notice may make physicians unwilling to come to the committee in the absence of overt disagreement between the physician and the patient. Giving notice to patients may cause them considerable distress, for no particular gain, if they are not party to a disagreement. Other questions punctuate this issue: Who is to notify the patient? If a case is referred anonymously or by a nurse, social worker, or other nonphysician, who gives the notice? What if the physician objects? Surely, in some of these cases, giving notice could make matters worse for the patient—at least in the short run.

We believe that patients should, in general, be informed if their case is to be reviewed by an ethics committee. That is, it is presumed that the patient will be notified unless there is some important reason not to give notice. A decision *not* to inform patients requires specific justification, which should be recorded in the committee's records of the review. When there is active, clearly expressed disagreement between the doctor and the patient or family, notice is essential so that the patient and family can present their views if they wish to do so.

When the disagreement is between members of the health care team, the question becomes more difficult. If the committee's policy is to write notes in the patient's chart, then the committee should remember that in many states patients have legal access to their charts. For further discussion of this problem, see chapter 11, "Privacy, Confidentiality, and Privilege."

Additional problems can arise when cases are referred anonymously. The committee may choose not to consider anonymously referred cases, but in some hospitals, lower echelon staff may reasonably fear the results of even minimal "whistle-blowing." Handling these cases requires considerable tact, and the committee should consider both the benefits and the risks of giving notice to the primary physician and the treatment team of anonymous referrals. The ethics committee may want to designate one member to conduct a preliminary review of such a case before the committee decides to take an official position on review. There is great diversity in notification and review participation practices, but ethics committees should be counseled not to operate so discretely that their reviews take on the look of secret trials or conspiracies.

Must Reviews Be Conducted by the Entire Committee?

Some committees will not review a case unless a quorum is present. These committees have decided that the need for group consideration is greater than the need to be able to respond quickly to requests for review. Other committees designate specific members to field requests and to handle them as they think best, involving other committee members as needed along the way. If the designated committee member thinks the case needs review by the entire ethics committee, then either a prompt meeting is called or, if possible, the case is held over to the next regular meeting.

Just as case review ought not to be the first activity that an ethics committee undertakes, independent actions by committee members ought not to be a starting point. Increased understanding about how to conduct reviews and about how the committee members respond to specific situations will develop over time during whole-committee reviews. A considerable degree of mutual trust is required for the entire committee to permit one or two members to act in its name. Developing that trust and mutual respect takes time. However, when that stage has been reached, the ethics committee can provide better service to the hospital by being more responsive to the actual needs. It may be psychologically difficult for committee members to fail to respond to all requests, but they should remember that it is better to do too little well than to do too much poorly.

How Are Case Reviews Concluded?

The conclusion of a case review might be a specific recommendation, the approval of a range of options, one or more suggestions, or a summary of the advantages and disadvantages of the alternatives. All cases that come before the committee need not have the same type of conclusion, but the ethics committee should be aware of why it has decided to handle a review in one way or another. Some committees are consistent insofar as they never provide a recommendation or, alternatively, always conclude a review with a statement of the committee's consensus about what actions are appropriate. Some writers have suggested that, with respect to case review, the ethics committee's primary function is to ensure that any proposed decision by physician or patient surrogate falls within the ethically acceptable range of treatment options. With this understanding of purpose, a committee might fall short of making recommendations, but still go further than simply discussing options.

Committees that refuse to make recommendations usually do so because they think that recommendations are actually the first step toward making treatment decisions and they do not wish to enter that territory. Committees that always make a consensus statement may be concerned about the need for some kind of closure so that both those who refer cases and the committee members themselves know what they have done and what, if anything, is to be done next. Committees that make neither recommendations nor suggestions are likely to be very informally structured committees that are offering case review as a discussion forum, using the cases to help everyone become better educated about the issues. As a result, its members are less likely to think that the case reviews are too amorphous and indecisive if some specific recommendation is not given. If the purpose is general education, then a specific recommendation is not needed (although the person who brought the case to the committee should be advised beforehand that no specific recommendations are likely to be forthcoming). This points out the need for the ethics committee to be very clear about the purpose of conducting case reviews (either in general or with respect to particular cases). It is easier to understand what should happen at the conclusion of the case review if the committee is clear about the reasons for doing the review at all.

Similarly, questions about whether votes should be taken, whether consensus is appropriate (and how consensus is determined), whether decisions should be recorded, and whether chart notations should be made depend upon how the ethics committee perceives its role. Decisions regarding chart notations may also depend upon the hospital's policy. (For a discussion of voting and for additional discussion of chart notations, see chapter 7.) Each committee must address these questions specifically. The committee may not want to make general rules about any of these matters, deciding instead to assess what is necessary or appropriate in cases as they arise. It should be noted that even if the ethics committee decides, for example, that it wants to make a chart notation stating that a case review was conducted and that a specific recommendation was made, it may also have to decide whether the committee chairman or the attending physician is to make that notation. Most committees do not make chart notations at this time, although they do make recommendations, take votes, and keep specific records of both.

Retrospective Review

Retrospective review differs considerably from *prospective review*. In general, prospective reviews look at the available options in a single case and retrospective reviews look at a group of cases *as a class*. Some writers have suggested that, if a committee intends to carry out prospective case reviews, it would be well advised to begin with retrospective reviews in order to ensure that the members have the necessary skills. Others have suggested that retrospective review is an appropriate committee function because it will enable members to identify the kinds of clinical situations in their hospital that require new policies or guidelines. Both of these reasons make sense, but we know of no committees at this time that are doing retrospective review routinely (that is, as a form of mandatory case review). Many committees, of course, use previous cases from their hospital experience rather than hypothetical cases for the purpose of committee education.

Conducting retrospective reviews would usually require that the committee decide to look at all cases of a certain kind. The most commonly suggested are cases in which newborns have had treatment withheld or withdrawn, cases in which adult incompetent patients have had life-prolonging treatment withheld, and cases in which DNR orders are written. The 1985 Baby Doe regulations suggest that infant care review

committees retrospectively review all cases in which infants had treatment withheld, unless the case had been reviewed prospectively by the committee. Interest in retrospective review may increase if prospective review is not conducted and if there are cases of clear abuse of decision-making power.

If a committee chooses to conduct retrospective reviews, it should have clear authorization to do so from the hospital administration, the governing board, or the medical executive committee. A mechanism should be in place for the committee to be informed about cases that fall within the class of interest. The committee will need to inform hospital physicians and employees of the kind of case it is reviewing, why it is reviewing these cases, and what it will do with the information gained in the process. Retrospective review has the potential for creating considerable hostility, because it may appear that the committee is looking over the physicians' shoulders and "second guessing" their decisions and actions. Because of this potential, education using retrospective review should stress that the purpose is not to fault actions in particular cases but only to see whether there are problems that could be handled more effectively if there were better policies or guidelines in place.

When retrospective reviews *are* requested for individual cases (instead of for a class of cases), the committee should be very cautious. A family member, a patient, a nurse, or a social worker might request that the ethics committee review a specific case after the fact. If the case is used simply as an exercise in committee education, there is no problem. If, however, the person who brings the case to the committee expects something more, the committee should consider whether or not it wants to address the issue, asking itself what the function of review is in such a case. The committee should try not to be drawn into disputes between individuals who are looking for someone to be found in error. It is possible that retrospective review of an individual case may give the committee some sense of a general problem. If it will not, however, then the committee should hesitate to take on such a review.

Retrospective review may also result in a conflict of issue jurisdiction with quality assurance or risk management committees. Before undertaking retrospective reviews, a committee would be well advised to consult with other appropriate hospital committees. It is possible that these reviews could be conducted jointly or that the reviewing would be the work of one committee and the policy making the work of another committee.

Retrospective review can give a committee an understanding of problems that it would not otherwise hear about, but it should not be a simple fishing expedition for problems. Without any indication that the handling of a particular kind of case is problematic, the committee might leave well enough alone. However, when committee members have heard anecdotal information about problems, retrospective review might be a reasonable way to find out if there are problems that need attention. Retrospective review could sometimes be combined with evaluation. For example, in determining the effectiveness of a DNR policy, a committee could conduct a retrospective review of all cases involving DNR orders.

Notes

1. Fost, N., and Cranford, R. E. Hospital ethics committees: Administrative aspects. *JAMA.* 1985. 253(18):2687-92.

2. Purtillo, R. Ethics consultations in the hospital. *N Engl J Med.* 1984. 311(15):983-6; Basson, M. Bioethics in the medical center. *Hosp Practice.* 1984 July. 19(7):177.

References

American Hospital Association. *Developing policies and procedures for long-term care institutions.* Chicago: AHA, 1975.

Bayley, C., and Cranford, R. E. Techniques for committee self-education and institution-wide education. In: Cranford and Doudera, eds. *Institutional Ethics Committees.* Ann Arbor, MI: Health Administration Press, 1984, pp. 149-56.

Capron, A. M. Decision review: a problematic task. In: Cranford and Doudera, eds. *Institutional Ethics Committee.*Ann Arbor, MI: Health Administration Press, 1984, pp. 174-85.

Gekas, B. G., and Countryman, K. M. *Development and Implementation of a Patient's Bill of Rights in Hospitals.* Chicago: AHA, 1980.

Jonsen, A., Siegler, M., and Winslade, W. J. *Clinical Ethics.* New York: Mcmillan Co., 1982.

Levine, C., and Veatch, R. M. eds. *Cases in Bioethics.* Hastings-on Hudson, New York: Hastings Center, 1982.

Levine, M. D., Scott, L., and Curran, W. J. Ethics rounds in a children's medical Center. *Pediatrics.* 1977. 60:202-8.

Macklin, R. Consultative roles and responsibilities. In: Cranford and Doudera, eds. *Institutional Ethics Committees.* Ann Arbor, MI: Health Administration Press, 1984, pp.157-68.

Mazonson, P. D., Gibson, J. M., and Saiki, J. H. Medical ethics rounds: development and organization. *Rocky Mountain Medical Journal.* 1979. 76(6):282-8.

Rothenberg, L. S. Guidelines for decision making: ethical values and limitations. In: Cranford and Doudera, eds., *Institutional Ethics Committees.* Ann Arbor, MI: Health Administration Press, 1984, pp.169-73.

Shannon, T. A. *What guidance from guidelines? Hastings Cent Rep.* 1977. 7(3):28-30.

Stalder, G. Ethical committees in a pediatric hospital. *Eur J Pediatr* 1981. 136(2):119-22.

Chapter 9

Problems and Pitfalls
for Ethics Committees

Many people have written about why the ethics committee is a good or a bad idea. Those who are critical believe that the potential for problems is greater than the potential for good. Despite criticism and hesitation on the part of many, ethics committees are being formed with increasing frequency in hospitals throughout the country. Many of the advance criticisms can stand as useful warnings, however, and in this section we will discuss some of those warnings. If the committee members realize that these problems are probably inherent, they will be able to anticipate them and deal with them more effectively.

Lack of Clarity
in Committee Purpose

An ethics committee's purpose stands in relation to its functions as a policy's principles stand in relation to its procedures. It is easy, in both cases, to forget the higher statement and focus solely on the more direct, action-oriented material. Sometimes, committees have no sense of their purpose because they have never considered it. It is certainly possible for a committee to operate without any genuine understanding of why it exists. For some ethics committees, the purpose seems obvious and thus does not need to be discussed. Yet, there is no generally agreed upon purpose for medical ethics committees. Expediency alone is not a sufficient purpose, and no law requires hospitals to have committees.

A committee may serve more than one purpose, of course, but it should have a primary purpose. If ethics committee members do not know the primary purpose of their committee's existence, they are likely to assume a purpose. If they do not agree about the purpose (either explicitly stated or tacitly assumed), members are likely to be frustrated and confused when what they perceive as the purpose does not seem to correspond with the actions of the committee. A member who believes that the committee exists to ensure specific ethical practices may be hard-pressed in consultation to deal with the member who thinks the committee exists to give health care providers a place to think out loud. A member who incorrectly believes that the committee's purpose is to open up more options in treatment decisions (when in fact the committee exists primarily to recommend policies and guidelines) will be hard-pressed to understand why the committee spends all its time talking about what should be done generally, rather than specifically.

When established, the committee should have a written statement of its purpose and overall goals. These may be supplied by the medical executive committee, the administration, the governing board, or the task force (depending upon how the ethics committee came into existence). In some cases, the ethics committee itself may be asked to develop a statement of its purpose and functions. Verbal statements alone are risky because they are open to interpretation over time. The meaning and importance of the written purpose should be impressed upon new members. Members of long standing may be so familiar with the purpose that they may neglect to explain it to new members, assuming that it is obvious.

A committee would be wise to establish specific goals at intervals of six months to one year, discussing how these short-term goals meet the committee's overall goals and serve the committee's purpose. By this means, the committee will regularly examine and be mindful of its purpose.

Predominance of the Case Review Function

College and university teachers have long known that students rate bioethics courses very highly, even if they are poorly taught, because the material is inherently interesting. The same phenomenon can occur with ethics committees—some activities are more interesting than others. Compared to case consultation, discussing and writing policies and guidelines, as well as providing education, can be extremely frustrating, seeming to yield little or no result. Progress is slow and disagreements often seem to arise from petty and irrelevant considerations. When it takes over a year to write and gain approval for a single policy (which is not uncommon), committee members may well feel that the cost-benefit ratio for such work is poor. Consultation, on the other hand, is more dramatic, faster, and more attuned to one's expectations of providing a successful intervention or genuine help. Health care workers' training and professional socialization emphasize active intervention, not consideration, reflection, and delay. Furthermore, the nature of their work tends to be such that they receive rapid feedback about the effect of their interventions. They are likely to see more passive activities (like policy writing) as meaningless or as "getting bogged down in procedures."

This conflict can create a serious problem. Many writers have feared that committees might gravitate toward case consultations as their primary activity. (In 1984, our initial survey of ethics committees in Catholic hospitals in California indicated that many new committees do begin their work with case consultation.) Such an emphasis surely heightens the risk that decision making will be perceived as being transferred from the doctor-patient relationship in the clinical setting to the ethics committee. The very fact that ethics committees make recommendations increases the pressure on the physician to accede to their judgment (rather than to his or her own) because of the assumed legal implications of ignoring the recommendation.

As many persons have pointed out, committee members learn about ethics and ethical decision making very effectively through either actual or hypothetical case discussions, and case reviews are used regularly for that purpose. Prospective review, however, is a very risky way to educate. The committee should be well educated *before* it begins conducting prospective case reviews. Retrospective review and review of hypothetical cases are less risky educational modes than prospective case reviews and can help members to better understand one another's perspectives and concerns. Using them may also help to meet committee members' needs for more active involvement. However, unless the committee's primary purpose is to be involved in the decision making process, members should be helped to understand that the primary work of the committee (education and policy recommendation) will be slow, not very dramatic, and sometimes very obscure in its effects. Furthermore, the development of good policies and effective education programs should prevent some problems and reduce the need for case consultation.

In addition, the committee may lack a sense of its own style or it may be changing its style. Committees might want to consider directly whether they should go out and find issues or wait for the issues to come to them, whether they should develop overall strategies or simply provide options for specific problems as they arise. If consultation is overemphasized, overall strategies for dealing with ethical problems of clinical care are likely to be lacking, although overall strategies are much more likely to make an important difference in the hospital's ethical awareness. Again, however, the primary orientation of health care and health care professionals may affect the choices that the ethics committee makes.

Contemporary American health care is oriented toward intervening in existing illness rather than in preventing illness. This attitude is characterized by a tendency to wait for problems to arise and find their way to the committee before deciding how such problems should be handled. Thus, for example, a committee might choose not to discuss whether it should establish policy or procedures regarding how to respond to requests from patients to the committee. Instead, the committee would assume that only when it receives such a request and understands its unique nature will the committee be able to decide how it should respond to the request. This style may dominate the ethics committee's functions without its members being aware that they have chosen one style over another. This style is surely a legitimate approach and, because the style is more familiar, it may make the committee's work more interesting and enjoyable. Nevertheless, it is probably less efficient.

Insufficient Member Education

Ethics committees cannot expect to educate others until they have first educated themselves. Educating members of ethics committees is an ongoing process, but members typically have inadequate time to gain a thorough grounding in the field. New members will, for the most part, be unfamiliar with the language of ethics and law, with relevant legal cases, and even with current controversies. If they are to be effective, they will have to undertake considerable self-study. Recently, however, many ethics committees have been created (some very precipitously) in the wake of the Baby Doe legislation and regulations, thereby intensifying the problem of educating new committee members. In the past, new committees have had the luxury of taking a year or more simply to educate themselves. Only when they felt they were ready did they begin to provide case reviews or to address the hospital's needs for new policies and education. Nowadays, a committee can find that at their very first meeting they are asked to deal with a difficult clinical dilemma.

Committees need to realize that taking action of any kind before their members feel competent is likely to cause more harm than good. Although a current problem may seem extremely demanding, the committee must keep in mind that such problems existed before the committee was appointed and that the hospital has methods of handling them. Perhaps the hospital's methods are not as sophisticated or effective as the ethics committee's methods will be when the members are ready, but they are also not impossible. A committee that gets in too deep needs to draw back, to set realistic boundaries of what it can and cannot do at any specific time in its development. Some suggest that subcommittees of the group can undertake activities that would be impossible for the larger group. This might be particularly attractive if some members of the committee have more experience with ethics problems. However, the danger of this practice is that the subgroup will be speaking for the entire committee before the committee knows what it has to say. In general, before a subcommittee is delegated to handle specific material (especially case reviews), the entire committee should have undertaken the activity so that everyone on the committee understands the boundaries of committee standards and the core of committee values.

When a committee has operated over a longer period of time and takes in a number of new members, there may be a tendency to expect the new members to pick up their knowledge on the run. Certainly there cannot be a long period of education each time new members are taken onto the committee. Committees should, however, provide one or two orientation periods for new members, making sure that they understand basic information about the committee's purpose, goals, prior activities, operating rules, and the nature of ethics in clinical care. New members should be given adequate written information to help them to understand how the committee functions and what is expected of them. Beyond that, committees may want to create some kind of "buddy system" by which each new member is paired with an experienced member. The old member's responsibility would be to help the new member develop necessary competence, to suggest additional resources for further education, and to make sure the new member is effectively integrated into the committee. After the first few months on the committee, new members should be asked specifically whether they feel able to participate fully in meetings or whether they need some further help to become sufficiently well-educated.

Enthusiasm and Frustration

Committee members often bring to the committee a shortage of time and an abundance of enthusiasm. This combination can create problems, although it is certainly preferable to an abundance of time and a shortage of enthusiasm! The enthusiasm may lead to elaborate plans; the time constraints may lead to little accomplishment. The result may be a feeling of frustration. Establishing realistic goals is vitally important for the committee and should be the special concern of the committee chairman. If the committee has taken on more than it can do, it should acknowledge its limitations and retrench. Otherwise, many of the committee's enthusiastic plans will simply drift into the middle distance, never to be heard of again. Persons who were interested in the particular goals that have been silently abandoned may feel that they themselves are being slighted. Many people have talked about committees providing education, consultation, and policy recommendation, though no one has explained how that is supposed to be achieved in 90 to 120 minutes per month.

If attendance begins to be very sporadic, members begin to forget about subcommittee meetings, meetings seem to wander over many topics but produce no plans or products (even paper ones), and it is difficult to find volunteers for committee projects, something may have gone awry. Such situations will probably not improve unless the problem is addressed directly. A sense of direction and the presence of reachable goals are both vital for ethics committees. If the direction does not exist, it cannot shape committee meetings or members' expectations. If the goals do not exist, then members will not know why they are attending meetings.

Hierarchy and Domination

The hospital is an institution with a strong sense of hierarchy. It is difficult to leave that hierarchy outside the doors of the committee's meeting room. A committee has hierarchy problems if a physician must be or always is the chairman (unless the committee's administrative structure requires a physician to be chairman); if only the physicians express disagreement; if the nurses do not offer their opinions on anything of importance or if their opinions are never solicited; if the lay members or nonhospital community members never speak or if when they speak they are listened to politely, but effectively ignored; or if disagreements are frequently halted by charges that some persons do not understand the medical situation. Hierarchy problems can manifest themselves in other ways as well.

No matter what the official purpose of the ethics committee may be, one of the underlying assumptions about ethics committees is that they provide a forum for discussing different values. Different values can be considered only if the people who hold them and who do not usually have a hospital forum for expressing them are willing and able to speak up. The hierarchy problem is not so much one of doctors refusing to listen to others as it is of others deferring to physicians' opinions. Sometimes, reticent members should be asked to voice their opinions and to give their judgments before the more dominant committee members speak. Otherwise, they may simply agree with what has already been expressed. Furthermore, their contributions to the discussion, even if not accepted as a final decision, should be acknowledged as useful and meaningful.

Many ethics committees depend upon consensus rather than upon formal voting procedures for decisions. The problem with the consensus approach is that members' deference to dominant or hierarchically superior members is easily obscured. This can also occur, of course, when formal votes are called if voice vote alone is used. If the chairman believes that some members of the committee are being excessively deferential, it may be advisable, again, to solicit their opinions specifically in order to determine whether committee decisions are, in fact, being made by consensus or, instead, by dominant professionals or personalities.

Inadequate Resources

In many hospitals, ethics committees operate with few or no resources other than the members themselves. Meetings may be held in off-hours, in which case both physicians and staff must volunteer their time. Especially when the members are contributing their own time, that contribution must be acknow-

ledged by the hospital in the form of appropriate support services to the committee. Furthermore, if the hospital believes that the committee should exist, then it has an obligation to provide it with enough resources (both dollars and staff time) to do its expected work. At a minimum, clerical assistance must be provided. Beyond that, there should be some discretionary funds for educational purposes (attending ethics conferences; subscribing to ethics journals, newsletters, and so forth; renting audiovisual materials; producing education programs for the community; and paying speakers who present special information to the committee).

Some committees have a staff person, part of whose job is to work with the committee. If a committee has such a staff person, it is preferable to have one who has the interest and capacity to deal with the substantive issues of the committee's work. Although some of the support work is strictly clerical, other work that needs to be done (screening the literature and setting up educational conferences, for example) requires a broader understanding.

Committee Overlap

Committee members need to be sensitive to the potential overlaps between ethics committees and other hospital committees that also deal with ethical issues in clinical care. Institutional review boards (IRBs), quality assurance (sometimes called quality review or quality care) committees, risk management committees, and utilization review committees all may be aware of cases or problems that need to come to the attention of the ethics committee. Similarly, issues that come to the ethics committee may need to be referred to or discussed with one of these other hospital committees.

Institutional review boards are required by federal law to review all research protocols using or intending to use any federal funds. Although IRB review is not legally required for all research, most institutions have policies requiring that all research, regardless of funding sources, be reviewed and approved by the institutional IRB before the project is begun. For the most part, IRBs review informed consent documents and ensure that the risks and benefits of the research protocol are appropriately balanced and that potential subjects will be properly informed about the research project.

Ethics committees might be asked to review cases involving patients in research projects if, for example, a staff member believes that one or more patients are not being given adequate or correct information on which to base their choices, even though the IRB-approved form is adequate. A patient who is refused participation in a research project might also come to an ethics committee. It is impossible to make any definitive statements about which ethical problems in research protocols "belong" to ethics committees and which "belong" to the IRB. In some facilities, the IRB and ethics committee are one and the same. In most hospitals and medical centers, however, they are separate. We believe that it is better to separate these two groups, first because the workload of each is substantial, and second because the tasks are quite different.

When they are separate groups, ethics committees would be well advised to be sure that their hospital IRB knows of their existence. Whenever a case comes to their attention that involves research, the ethics committee should inform the IRB and a joint decision made about which group should handle it. If the hospital has considerable research, the ethics committee and the IRB should develop a close relationship and consider either having one or two members in common or appointing liaisons from each group to the other.

Quality review, quality care, or quality assurance committees are medical staff committees that are intended to ensure overall quality of care in the hospital. They generally receive referrals from specialty groups (department committees) and are not usually concerned with individual cases. Quality review committees ordinarily review practices and, when quality of care problems become apparent, write policies or guidelines to reduce or eliminate those problems. A quality review committee might request an ethics committee to prepare a policy in an area that involved primarily ethical problems rather than primarily medical issues. Medical and ethical problems often coexist and are frequently confused. The ethics committee should carefully consider whether a case it receives for review involves medical or ethical issues and, if the case is primarily medical, should refer the matter to the quality review committee (or, at least, discuss whether referral is appropriate).

Some persons believe that, because *quality of care* is a more general term than *ethics,* both ethical and medical issues should come before the quality review committee. We do not believe both functions should be carried out by a single committee even though conflicts concerning referrals may occur when there are separate committees. "Turf-fighting" cannot be helpful to anyone, and the ethics committee, as the newer group, should take care to inform the quality review committee of the work the ethics group is undertaking and how it complements the activities of the quality review committee.

Utilization review committees direct the activities of the utilization review department, monitor resources used by the hospital, and review cases for determining proper use of the facilities (for example, bed use, patient length of stay, services ordered, and so forth). They customarily draw the attention of the medical staff and the administration to problems of resource allocation and make recommendations about future trends. In the past, the utilization review committee has been concerned about overuse of the amount of medical care and the length of hospitalization necessary for patients; in the future, these groups may need to be concerned with *underuse* because of DRGs.

To the extent that ethics committees are involved in allocation or rationing decisions, their work may overlap with the utilization review committee. Utilization review committee recommendations should reflect appropriate ethical considerations, especially when resources are being rationed rather than allocated. (For an explanation of this distinction, see "Allocation of Resources," in chapter 3.) In a new economic climate, utilization review recommendations may shift from whether the insurance company will pay to whether anticipated benefits justify specific forms of treatment. The ethics committee may want to provide education programs for persons who make allocation or rationing decisions in order to ensure that they consider the ethical dimensions, as well as the cost-benefit ratio, of this type of decision.

Because *risk management committees* are particularly concerned with questions of legal liability (malpractice as well as general concerns with patient safety), their functions, too, may overlap those of the ethics committee, insofar as legal and ethical issues overlap. Risk management committees have not, however, taken a significant role in developing ethics committees in most hospitals. When both committees exist in a facility, there may be a tendency to treat law and ethics as if they were mutually exclusive concerns.

Arguments exist both for and against including risk managers as members of ethics committees. Official membership on the committee ensures better communication between the two groups and reduces the likelihood of rigid separation of law and ethics. On the other hand, risk managers are frequently the official liaison with the hospital attorney. The arguments against having hospital attorneys as committee members can also apply to risk managers because they, too, may have a conflict of interest. If they perceive their responsibility as reducing legal liability, then they may have difficulty accepting ethically appropriate actions that have the necessary consequence of increasing the risk of liability or the risk of litigation. (For further discussion of hospital attorneys as committee members, see the "Lawyers" section in chapter 6.)

Ideally, the committees should work cooperatively, informing one another of situations with both legal and ethical dimensions. Ethics committees should always inform risk management whenever any action they take — in specific cases or as matters of policy — could increase the hospital's risk of liability.

Evaluation Failures

Most committees fail to evaluate the work they have done. Indeed, given the constraints of time, evaluation may seem an extraordinary luxury. Nevertheless, both formal and informal evaluations should be conducted regularly. If they are not, the committee can easily lose track of what it is doing and how well it is doing it.

There are many ways to evaluate the committee's work and its effectiveness. Though frequently used, the intuitive approach is not adequate. Evaluation forms are common at conferences and education meetings. Evaluation makes it possible for those who are responsible for organization and planning to determine whether or not they are successful. Administration (and committees are a form of administration) is at its best when it exists to make work on the front lines more effective and more rewarding. It is when committees (as well as other administrators) fail to check whether they are making their colleagues' work easier or harder, more or less effective, that they fall from good administration to bad bureaucracy.

Because so little is known about how groups like ethics committees can work effectively in the hospital, it is imperative for committees to reflect and to investigate on a regular basis to see how they are doing. Everyone would, of course, prefer to be doing well and to be doing more of what they are already comfortable doing. Nevertheless, no one is likely to be doing perfectly when the venture is new and the team is untested.

A failure to evaluate the effects of its work may lead to the committee's becoming isolated in the hospital community. A failure to evaluate the committee members' own sense of and satisfaction with their role can be equally destructive to the committee's long-term success. If the committee becomes known as do-nothing, argumentative, dominating, top-heavy, or intolerant, enthusiastic and knowledgeable new members will be hard to find. The committee will become the home of those who have nothing better to do.

This section on potential problem areas for committees began with a discussion of the importance of the committee understanding its purpose. It ends with an insistence upon the importance of regular evaluation. These two go hand in hand. Evaluation permits the members to judge whether they are furthering the committee's purpose and whether they are doing it effectively. (For additional discussion of evaluation, see "Committee Evaluation," in chapter 7, as well as appendix E.)

Reference

McCormick, R. A. Ethics committees: promise or peril? *Law, Med Health Care.* 1984. 12(4):150-5.

Part III

Legal Issues
for Bioethics Committees

Chapter 10

How the Legal System Works

Although it is not the ethics committee's responsibility to assess legal concerns, committee members should have a general knowledge of the way in which legal requirements impinge upon clinical health care decisions. In addition, they need specific knowledge of the legal reasoning upon which some court decisions are based. The following chapters attempt to provide that background through brief discriptions of the way in which courts operate and of specific decisions.

Law and Ethics

Legal issues and ethical issues in health care often seem inextricably intertwined because United States law embodies some but not all aspects of the moral standards of our culture. The relationship between law and ethics is complex. Some writers have suggested that, in most instances, law represents a culture's minimum ethical standard; others have argued that the distinction is greater, for everything legal is not necessarily moral and vice versa. In the United States, where there are many different subcultures and a national commitment to pluralistic values, both these statements seem to say something accurate about the relationship between law and ethics. It is important to remember, however, that law and ethics are not interchangeable, that is, establishing the legality of an action does not speak to its morality. Health care professionals and institutions, especially hospitals operated by religious groups, are likely to establish and abide by ethical standards of care that are more demanding than the minimum standards required by law.

Legal standards alone fail to provide adequate ethical guidance for other reasons, as well. Law usually moves behind social practices and the development of law requires a conflict or a disagreement about how something should be done. That is, legal questions and their resolutions do not usually arise until after the actions or behaviors that embody the questions have taken place and someone disagrees with them. For example, until surrogate parenting contracts were actually being made (and were breaking down), no one questioned how the law should address the problem, nor how statutes should be drawn up. Furthermore, in such cases, what was clearly a moral question could not be answered by any preexisting, straightforward, legal standard or rule.

In matters involving novel conflicts (and bioethics issues are for the most part new problems), the law initially attempts to use previous rulings about similar situations to determine what is appropriate. When the situations are not sufficiently similar, then courts and legislators throughout the country are likely to provide either no answers or several differing answers about what is "legal." This difference of standards disconcerts persons who believe that law should say what is right and frustrates those who must make decisions without clearly defined or consistent legal criteria. Frequently, when there are different versions of statutes across the country, the American Law Institute or the National Conference of Commissioners on Uniform State Laws will propose what is called a *model uniform law*. States will then frequently adopt that version of the law. This has happened with brain-death statutes, which once varied widely, and many states have adopted the model uniform law version.

Law as a standard has its limitations. Yet, despite its inconsistencies and lack of clarity, law is essential simply because it binds us together as a *civic* community. Law exists in several forms: *statutory law,* from statutes passed by elected representatives (city councils, county supervisors, state legislatures, or the U.S. Congress); *regulatory law,* from regulations established by government agencies; and *case law,* from federal and state court decisions. For the most part, statutory laws that relate to ethical problems in clinical health care are passed at the state level. Similarly, most court decisions on these issues will and do emanate from the state court system. Ethics committees need to know the relevant regulatory and statutory law in their own geographic region, the court decisions that are legally binding upon medical decision making in their state or region, and the decisions made in other states and districts that are likely to influence local courts. In addition, they need to understand how the judicial system works so that they can appreciate the meaning and effect of court decisions at every level.

Structure of the Judicial System

The following description of the United States court system is brief and general. In any complex institutional system, many exceptions to the general patterns exist. We have not attempted to note exceptions here, nor have we made regular distinctions between criminal law and civil law. The reader should be reminded that all *general* statements are, to a degree, inaccurate.

The United States has two court systems: state courts and federal courts. The two systems are generally separate: matters involving state laws are usually tried within the state system and matters involving federal laws are usually tried within the federal system. A state matter can cross over into the federal system, however, if there are claims involving violations of constitutional rights. Such matters first go through the state system (including the state supreme court) and then can be appealed to the U.S. Supreme Court in the federal system.

The State Court System

The state court system has three levels: *municipal* and *superior* courts, *state appellate* courts, and *state supreme* courts. Some states use different nomenclature so that a *superior* court may be called a *supreme* court of the state. Whatever the name used by the particular state, the functions at each level remain the same.

At the first state level, *municipal and superior courts* function as trial courts. They hear the facts that each side alleges to be true and they apply the appropriate laws. A jury or a judge may decide the case, depending upon a number of factors. Only one judge hears the case and the judge seldom provides a written decision at the trial level. If the plaintiff or defendant in a civil case or the defendant in a criminal case is dissatisfied with the decision, he or she may appeal the decision to the appellate court and, in general, the appellate court must hear the case. (In criminal cases, appeals cannot be made if the defendant is found not guilty.)

Superior courts include felony criminal courts, mental health courts, juvenile courts, dependency courts, domestic relations courts, probate courts, and so forth. Municipal courts include traffic courts, misdemeanor criminal courts, small claims courts, justice of the peace courts, and so forth.

When a case is appealed to the second level in the state court system, it is heard by the *state appellate court* in that region. Each case is heard by a panel of three appellate justices from that region. The judges hear and decide the case together. Their decision may be unanimous or it may be split, but the majority decision rules. In general, state appellate courts take all cases submitted to them. Having heard a case, the appellate court may affirm the lower court ruling without giving any explanation for its decision or it may either agree or disagree with the lower court ruling but provide an extensive written opinion explaining its reasoning. In cases involving bioethics problems, the appellate courts are likely to give a written opinion because the decision has wide bearing and the situation will probably arise again. A written decision will usually clarify the actions that can and should be taken, under the circumstances, by patients, health care providers, hospital administrators, and so on.

The appellate courts do *not* hear cases *on the facts,* as do the trial courts. Appellate justices are expected to make their decisions solely on the basis of legal issues. That is, the question is not whether the judge or jury decided correctly about the *facts* that were presented at trial, but whether the *law* was applied correctly at the trial. After the appellate court gives its decision, the matter is ended if there is no subsequent appeal or if the case is not remanded (returned) to the lower court for retrial in light of the appellate decision. For example, the appellate court might find that a judge had instructed the jury incorrectly as to the meaning of specific legal terms and, thus, order the case to be tried again, this time using the correct instructions.

The decisions of the appellate court are binding upon all the superior and municipal courts within its region. That is, when the appellate court issues a written interpretation of a legal principle, the lower state courts within that region are obliged to accept it as the correct interpretation of the law. Appellate courts within the same state, however, are not bound by one another's decisions. As a result, what is legally permissible may vary between appellate regions within a state. When there is significant disagreement among the various courts, the state supreme court usually will agree to hear a case in the disputed area and make a decision that is henceforth binding on all the appellate and trial courts in that state. Decisions made in the courts of one state are not binding nor do they establish precedent for the courts of any other state. Nevertheless, justices usually pay attention to how other states are thinking about a specific problem. A state court decision can be very influential in other states if it is well-reasoned and/or well-received by the public and by the legal/professional community. The decision in the New Jersey *Quinlan* case, for example, has invariably been cited when other state courts decide terminating treatment cases.

If the plaintiff or defendant is not satisfied by the appellate court decision, he or she may appeal to the highest level of state court, usually called the *state supreme court*. Like the appellate court, the supreme court reviews lower court decisions, being concerned only with how the law was applied and interpreted, not with judging the facts of the case. The supreme court is not required to hear all cases that are appealed. Nor is it required to provide a written opinion if it does hear the case.

The court will take one of three possible actions when asked to hear a case. First, if it refuses to hear the case, then the appellate decision stands; moreover, although the appellate court's reasoning for the decision has not been officially accepted by the supreme court justices, there is a strong suggestion that they find it adequate. Second, if the supreme court does hear the case and if it affirms the lower court's judgment, then the supreme court has officially acknowledged the lower court's reasoning as correct.

Third, the supreme court may hear the appeal and produce (at one extreme) a single written opinion or (at the other extreme) one majority opinion, one or more concurring opinions, and one or more dissenting opinions. If either party is dissatisfied with the court's decision, he or she may, in some states, request the court to hear the case again. A state supreme court may rule on constitutional issues with regard to its own constitution. However, if the case involves a federal constitutional issue (for example, the appellant contends that the law in question violates the rights guaranteed to all citizens by the U.S. Constitution), then the case can be further appealed to the U.S. Supreme Court. A decision made by the state supreme court is binding on all lower state courts, but has no direct effect on federal courts at any level nor on the courts of other states.

Sometimes, judicial procedures occur even before a case goes to trial when there is a dispute about whether the action that is alleged against the defendant actually constitutes a legal wrong or injury. In such instances, the issue is whether there is or is not a legitimate *cause of action*. Cases involving disputes about the appropriateness of health care decisions sometimes involve questions of whether or not the case rests on a legitimate cause of action. People frequently confuse decisions about cause of action with decisions about the guilt, innocence, or liability of the defendants. Two important cases, *Tarasoff*[1] and *Barber-Nejdl*,[2] involve cause-of-action decisions, but are often discussed as if they involved findings of innocence or nonliability. The California Appellate Court decisions in these cases are widely known among health care professionals, but frequently it is thought that the therapist in the *Tarasoff* case was found "guilty" and that Doctors Barber and Nejdl were found "innocent." In fact, the *Tarasoff* case was never tried to determine whether the therapist had been negligent in failing to warn the Tarasoff family of the threat to their daughter's life. Nor was there ever a trial to determine whether Doctors Nejdl and Barber were guilty or innocent of homicide. Rather, the decisions in these two cases (both cases had more than one decision) were concerned with whether or not there was a cause of action against the defendants.

A case can be heard by a trial court only if there is a legally recognized conflict, that is, an appropriate cause of action. The law recognizes that all citizens have certain "general" duties toward one another. In addition, professionals have special duties toward their clients or patients. In both *Tarasoff* and *Barber* there was a question of what the physician owed as a duty to the patient or the family. Thus, in the *Tarasoff* case, the question was whether a psychotherapist who fails to warn a threatened third person is behaving negligently; that is, do therapists have a legal duty to warn third persons who the therapists believed were at risk of being harmed by their patients? In the *Barber-Nejdl* case, the question was whether withdrawing ventilator, food, and fluids from a patient who was not brain-dead constitutes homicide as it is defined in the criminal code. The question was not whether the individuals did or did not do a specific act. In both cases, the physicians and the opposing parties agreed about what the physician had done. Instead, the question was whether or not the act that they had performed or failed to perform violated the law. In other words, an attorney might prove in court that the defendants had performed the alleged acts, but if those acts were not illegal, then it made no difference whether or not they did it. Thus, Doctors Nejdl and Barber were not acquitted or found innocent of the murder charges, as some people have said. Rather, the murder charges against them were dropped when the California Appellate court said that the actions with which the district attorney charged them did not constitute a homicide as defined by California law.

The Federal Court System

Federal courts, like state courts, are three-tiered. The first tier is made up of the *federal district courts*. The United States is divided into a number of regions, each of which has a federal district court. There is a district in each state and some states have more than one. The federal district courts, like state superior and municipal courts, are trial courts. They are the first to hear all cases involving federal statutes. Like state trial courts, a single judge presides over each court and cases may be decided either by judge or by jury.

In the federal system, the second tier is occupied by the *federal circuit courts*. Each of the 12 federal circuit courts (including Washington, DC) has a number of judges who hear cases in panels of three. There is a right of appeal from the district court; decisions are reviewed with respect to application and interpretation of law but not to the weighing of facts in evidence; and the justices are not required to give written decisions, although they do in many cases. The decisions of each circuit court are binding upon all the district courts that fall within that circuit. However, different circuit courts often make rulings that are inconsistent with one another on subjects about which the U.S. Supreme Court has not spoken. Decisions can be appealed to the U.S. Supreme Court, which may—or may not—choose to hear the case.

The *United States Supreme Court* is the highest court of the land. Its decisions are binding upon all federal courts and, with respect to interpretation of the Constitution and of federal statutes, upon all state courts as well. The U.S. Supreme Court has discretionary review over circuit court decisions: it may review lower court decisions if it chooses, but is not required to do so. It may review any decision by a state supreme court in which the appellant claims that his or her constitutional rights have been violated by the state. The disputed state action may be either a statutory law or a judicial decision interpreting law. If asked, the Court must review any state supreme court decision that upholds the validity of a state statute, although it can then dismiss the case for lack of a substantial federal question.

Historically, the states rather than the federal government have the authority to pass laws affecting domestic and other personal matters, including the doctor-patient relationship. As a result, most legal/ethical problems in health care come through the state courts rather than through the federal courts. The recent *Baby Jane Doe* case is an interesting example of a case that proceeded on different issues through both state and federal systems. The U.S. Supreme Court has decided few cases that directly address the issues customarily involved in bioethics, although, of course, many Supreme Court decisions have established important principles that relate to health care cases. Because the U.S. Supreme Court is the court of last appeal, it tends to wait until there has been substantial public discussion about the dimensions of a difficult issue before it agrees to hear a case. Although some courts have been more activist, the current U.S. Supreme Court is very willing to give the lower level courts ample opportunity to work out solutions before it becomes involved.

Constitutional Issues

The United States Constitution, including the Bill of Rights, defines and limits the relationship between individuals and the government, not the relationships between individuals. Thus, for constitutional issues to arise, the case must involve some kind of state or federal action. In assessing constitutional issues, the U.S. Supreme Court's function is not to address the wisdom, advisability, or goodness of a federal or state law or regulation. As Justice Stewart commented in his dissent in *Griswold v. Connecticut,*

> We are not asked in this case to say whether we think this law is unwise, or even asinine. We are asked [whether] it violates the United States Constitution. . . . It is the essence of judicial duty to subordinate our own personal views, our own ideas of what legislation is wise and what is not.

This accurately describes, at least in theory, the Court's function: the Court is to say only whether the Constitution, including the Bill of Rights, specifically forbids the states or the federal government to pass such a law or to establish such regulations. In practice, however, the U.S. Supreme Court has sometimes functioned as a super-legislature, displacing the judgments of state legislators about what constitutes an appropriate or wise law and putting forth their own view of the matter. The abortion decision *(Roe v. Wade)* is one example of a decision that reads more like legislation than constitutional interpretation. There are others, as well. The Court's willingness to make these "substantive due process decisions" has been more common in some periods than in others. Currently, the Berger court is somewhat less activist than the Warren court of the 1960s and 1970s. There are, however, objections from the legal and scholarly community each time the Court makes substantive due process decisions because the practice tends to blur the lines between the branches of government.

With respect to health care, the courts are likely to be addressing the constitutional issues of *privacy, freedom of religion,* and *equal protection.*

Privacy

The right of privacy was first announced by the Court in 1965 in *Griswold v. Connecticut,* a case involving a Connecticut state law forbidding the use of contraceptives. Several opinions were written in the case and the justices said that although the Constitution did not specifically mention any right of privacy, the right was implied. In the language of Justice William O. Douglas, the right of privacy "emanated" from "the penumbra" of the Bill of Rights. In this decision, the privacy that was being protected was that of the married couple. Douglas drew upon earlier cases involving parental rights to make decisions about child rearing practices. The decision was followed by others that also emphasized the important relationship between the right of privacy and family relationships.

Despite this tendency to identify constitutional privacy rights with marriage and family, the Court has not been very clear about exactly what it thinks is protected by the right of privacy. Lower courts (both lower federal courts and the state supreme courts) have all used the right of privacy to justify many different kinds of decisions, but at the present time there is no agreement about what privacy means or to what it applies. In the language of legal scholars, the "core concept" of privacy is unknown. Privacy is used by courts in three different senses: family privacy (matters relating to marital relationships or child rearing); an individual's right to avoid disclosure of personal matters (informational privacy); and an interest in independence or liberty for making certain kinds of important decisions that greatly influence an individual's sense of self (autonomy).

In bioethics literature, the right of privacy is frequently asserted as a justification for respecting individuals' decisions. That is, privacy rights are equated with the right of autonomy. For the most part, the U.S. Supreme Court has not been inclined to use the right of privacy in that sense, although other

courts have done so. When reading decisions based on or using privacy rights, one should make a distinction between whether the court is suggesting that the individual has an unfettered right to do something or whether it is asserting that a person has a right to make decisions in the context of a family or quasi-family situation. Decisions involving informational privacy are usually easily distinguished. The limits of the right of privacy as a means of protecting individual choices (that is, autonomy) is suggested by the Supreme Court's clear unwillingness to apply privacy right protection to sexual behavior between consenting adults of the same sex, for example.

Freedom of Religion

Freedom of religion lies within the first amendment protections. Because religions frequently have specific rules about medical practices, the courts have made rulings on the basis of constitutional implications of freedom of religion. In general, medical treatment cannot be forced upon any adult who wishes to refuse that treatment upon the basis of religious beliefs. Christian Scientists and Jehovah's Witnesses, two groups with well-known ideas about medical care, have sought and received constitutional protection for their refusal of standard medical care. The courts have not been sympathetic, however, to parents who claim a right to refuse treatment for their minor children on the basis of religious beliefs. In a 1944 case, *Prince v. Massachusetts,* the U.S. Supreme Court held that a state law designed to protect minors from exploitative labor was constitutional, even when it applied to a minor who was selling religious magazines on the street and even though the minor was in the custody of a relative. With respect to the religious freedom claimed by the defendant, the court replied that, while parents had a right to make martyrs of themselves, they had no right to make martyrs of their children. Using this decision, lower courts have regularly ordered medical treatment for children over their parents' religiously-motivated disapproval (and the child's disapproval as well) if the child's health would be seriously jeopardized without treatment.

Although the U.S. Supreme Court has not made any such decision, lower courts have also ordered medical treatment for parents of minor children in some cases when the parents have refused treatment for religious reasons. The courts' reasoning has been that it was necessary to override the religious freedom claim and to save the parent's life in order to protect the children who needed the parent. Health care cases involving freedom of religion claims may be growing more complex as a result of the proliferation of religious cults in America and the increasing concern about children's welfare in religious groups with unusual beliefs. (For a brief discussion of organized religions' attitudes toward specific health care practices, see appendix G.)

Equal Protection

Equal protection is the constitutional doctrine embodied in the 14th Amendment. Equal protection means that no state shall "deny to any person within its jurisdiction the equal protection of the laws." In its simplest form, equal protection forbids the state to pass laws that discriminate against any group unless there is a compelling reason to do so.

Equal protection claims have been made with respect to care for handicapped newborns. In the case of *Baby Jane Doe,* the government demanded access to the infant's hospital records in order to determine whether she was being denied equal protection. Their argument implied that she might not be receiving necessary medical treatment because she was mentally disabled. The U.S. Supreme Court did not rule on that case and the federal circuit court sidestepped the constitutional issue of equal protection by concluding that the cited federal law was not intended to cover situations like that of the infant. Thus, the constitutional issue was not reached.

The *Baby Jane Doe* Case: An Example of Court Procedures

On October 19, 1983, the U.S. Department of Health and Human Services (DHHS) received a complaint that an infant in the Stonybrook University Hospital, New York, was being denied medically indicated treatment on the basis of her handicap. The infant was reported to have spina bifida with hydrocephaly and microcephaly. (Later reports suggested that, contrary to press accounts, she was not microcephalic. Her head circumference, it was claimed, was well within the normal range of a child with spina bifida.) Lawrence Washburn, an attorney with no relation to the hospital, the physicians, or the baby's family, brought an action in a New York superior court, asking the court to appoint a temporary guardian for the infant and to consent to immediate surgery to close the spinal lesion and implant a shunt. Washburn's action alleged a violation of state law, in that parents have a duty to provide necessary medical care for their children. The trial court appointed a guardian and ordered surgery. The hospital appealed the order and the state appellate court reversed the lower court deci-

sion the next day. Washburn then appealed to the state supreme court. Some time later, the state supreme court affirmed the appellate court ruling, sharply commenting that the case should not have been brought in the first place because Washburn was not an interested party.

In the meantime, the federal government also took action. DHHS did not focus on parental duties (as did the state suit), but rather on questions of equal protection, that is, whether the baby was being subjected to unfair discrimination. In order to determine if there was a possibility of discrimination, the surgeon general sued the hospital in federal court for access to Baby Jane Doe's records. The hospital refused to release the records because they were confidential and protected by the infant's and family's rights of privacy. The federal district court ruled that the hospital did not have to turn over the records because it was clear from the state court record that the hospital was not discriminating against the infant—it was willing to perform the surgery. It had not done so because the parents had not given consent. The government appealed this decision to the federal circuit court of appeals, which affirmed the lower court decision and broadened it in a written opinion stating that the federal law forbidding discrimination against the handicapped (section 504 of that law was at issue) did not apply to treatment decisions for handicapped infants. The federal government chose not to appeal the decision to the U.S. Supreme Court.

The court actions in this case demonstrate how confusing individual cases can be. In this case, a single treatment decision generated two different and entirely separate court cases—one in the state system and one in the federal system—that were heard and decided during the same time period. Upon hearing about a decision, many people were very confused about which case the decision concerned. Others never realized that there were two different cases, with different plaintiffs and different decisions about different issues. The facts of the situation in both cases were accepted as those presented in the trial court at the state level. The appellate and supreme court decisions were concerned entirely with legal interpretation. This case was further confused by the fact that the second set of Baby Doe regulations, which apparently applied to Baby Jane Doe, were also being litigated in the federal courts throughout the same general time period. The decision on these regulations has now been appealed to the Supreme Court. The reader should note that the regulations and guidelines published by DHHS in 1985 as part of the 1984 amendments to the federal Child Abuse Prevention and

Treatment Program, and frequently referred to as *Baby Doe regulations* or *Baby Doe guidelines* are not the same regulations that the U.S. Supreme Court is hearing. The nomenclature in this instance serves only to add to the confusion.

Notes

1. The issue in the *Tarasoff* case was whether a psychotherapist had a duty to warn third parties if the therapist believed that his or her patient was likely to injure that third party. In this particular case, a therapist's patient had murdered a young woman with whom he was in love, and the therapist had known that such an action was on the patient's mind.

2. The *Barber-Nejdl* case involved the death of Clarence Herbert, a permanently unconscious patient. Mr. Herbert died after his ventilator and then I.V. lines were disconnected (with family consent), and Doctors Barber and Nejdl were charged with murder.

Chapter 11

Privacy, Confidentiality, and Privilege

Privacy, in the context of confidentiality, health care, and ethics committees, refers to the patient's control over his or her personal information. A patient's "right to privacy" refers (at least in this context) to the patient's right to keep personal information private. In seeking health care, the patient must both provide information and expose himself to many tests and observations. Thus, because the patient loses considerable control over his privacy, he is promised *confidentiality*.

Confidentiality is a legal and moral right derived from the right of privacy and reinforced by professional codes of ethics. With respect to informational privacy, confidentiality means that information is divulged by one person to another with the implicit promise that it will not be revealed to any other person. In the doctor-patient relationship, the patient reveals information about himself to a relative stranger (the physician) only because the physician needs that information to provide proper health care to the patient. The kind of information that patients reveal to physicians is highly personal; releasing their hold on this information makes patients vulnerable. Thus, the physician promises not to release the information to anyone else. (He or she will not "breach the confidentiality.") If the law requires that the physician reveal some kinds of patient information (for example, child abuse reporting), that is an exception to the duty to provide confidentiality, not a breach of confidentiality. If the patient requests that the information be released (for example, insurance reimbursement forms), that is a consented-to redisclosure, not a breach of confidentiality. Confidentiality, in the doctor-patient relationship, is breached only when information is released without a legal requirement to do so or without the patient's consent. The infor-

mation obtained in the doctor-patient relationship is always considered confidential. It may also be *privileged* if the state has granted it that status.

Privilege is a legally created right that is related to, but not identical to, confidentiality. Privilege (the word comes from the concept of privileged information) is granted by the state legislature; it denies courts and the legal process access to information about patients that professionals acquire as part of the doctor-patient relationship. The state can also make *exceptions* to the confidential status of information. Exceptions to confidentiality in the doctor-patient relationship may include requirements for reporting child abuse and abuse of the elderly, public health requirements to report communicable diseases, access to patient records for research, and others.

It should be noted that the claim of confidentiality lies with the patient or client, not with the professional. If the patient or client wishes confidential information released, then the professional must release it. If a patient or client does not want confidential information released, then the professional may not divulge it unless the state chooses to make some kind of exception.

Privacy and Confidentiality for the Patient

Confidentiality is a much cherished value in health care, and ethics committees that provide prospective or retrospective review of individual cases need to think about how the need for confidentiality applies to them. Confidentiality grows from concern for privacy rights so any question about confidentiality must first look to whose privacy is being protected and why.

Persons entering the health care system are required to give up some degree of privacy. They must give personal, private information about themselves to health care professionals as a condition of receiving medical care. Patients can claim a right of privacy for this information because losing control over that information may render them potentially vulnerable to harm, which can range from fear of embarrassment to physical harm. Because the disclosures are not voluntary—they are required as a condition of treatment—the patient can claim confidentiality. *Confidential* means *with faith,* that is, information is given with faith or with trust that the information will not be further disclosed without permission.

The claim to confidentiality is the patient's, not the physician's. The patient (the person who has been required to divulge private information, thus becoming vulnerable) has the *claim;* the person who has asked for the private information has the *duty* to see that the information does not go further, or does so only in very limited circumstances (such as to other health care professionals directly involved in the patient's treatment or as required by law). It is important to understand who has the *claim* for confidentiality because that is the person who can legitimately disclose information or permit others to disclose it.

The information that is protected by confidentiality in the doctor-patient relationship includes all information provided by the patient in the course of that relationship. A claim of confidentiality is all-encompassing. The physician or other health care professional is not permitted to judge whether the information is or is not potentially harmful and to reveal it if it is not. Strictly speaking, a decision to *redisclose* (that is, to tell someone other than the members of the health care team) is left to the patient's judgment. As a matter of practice, however, health care institutions make some kinds of distinctions about this. For example, hospitals are likely to give a telephone caller information about whether a specific person is a patient in the hospital and, if the caller says that he or she is a family member, are also likely to give limited information about the patient's condition. A mental hospital, however, is unlikely to do this and may be legally forbidden to provide any such information, even to family members, without specific permission from the patient, because being a patient in a mental hospital is potentially so stigmatizing. In either case, however, a patient could claim that the information was potentially harmful and if he or she had not given permission for the information to be released, the hospital could be said to have improperly violated the patient's expectations of confidentiality. Thus, as a general rule, all information that the patient

gives in the course of medical treatment should be assumed to be within the obligation of confidentiality and any decision to disclose it to someone else, if the disclosure is not legally required or consented to by the patient, is a breach of confidentiality and should be carefully considered.

Private information about patients is, of course, divulged to others in the course of treatment, but that is not considered a breach of confidentiality as long as the information is provided to others who are involved in the patient's care and treatment. With respect to confidentiality, the doctor-patient relationship is broadened to include nurses and social workers—all those who have a need to know private information about the patient in order to provide and to guarantee appropriate care.

The patient's claim to confidentiality may fall to legally required government reporting (for example, child abuse, elderly abuse, and venereal disease reports; tumor registers; and *Tarasoff* warnings). Whether or not patients should be routinely informed of such disclosures (either in advance or at the time the information is provided to the government or others) is vigorously debated. The patient may not forbid these reports, of course, but many writers believe that the nature of the doctor-patient relationship is such that the physician should inform the patient when such reports are made in order to honor the claims of confidentiality. (That is, the patient will be reassured by being informed when confidential information must be released, because he or she will understand that, in the absence of such notice, confidentiality is being maintained.) Others, however, believe that notifying patients of even the potential for such disclosures may be seen as too threatening and thus cause a loss of rapport between doctor and patient.

The second area in which disclosures are routinely made is to third-party payers, for which the patient is usually asked to give *blanket consent to disclosure.* In the confidentiality waivers that they require patients to sign, insurance companies frequently receive blanket permission for unspecified redisclosures. Although the moral appropriateness of blanket permissions and subsequent redisclosures (especially when specific notice is not given) is widely questioned, third party redisclosures always require some kind of patient consent, unless they are required by law.

Ethics Committees' Obligations of Confidentiality

Ethics committee members must think about how they fit into this schema. In cases of prospective consultations, committees usually receive extensive information that is normally held within the bounds of confidentiality. Often the patient is identified by name, but even if not, the patient's identity may be easily determined, especially in a hospital with an effective "grapevine." What is the committee's relationship to this patient? There are three ways to look at this: first, the committee can be included within the extended doctor-patient relationship, as are other members of the health care team, thus being bound by the same claims of confidentiality and of privilege as is the physician. Second, the committee may be seen to be like a medical staff committee, promoting overall patient care, thus being protected by whatever statutory privilege exists in the state and obligated by confidentiality claims. Third, it may be seen neither as a part of the doctor-patient relationship nor as a committee empowered to receive such information; if so, the committee may have no right to receive the information without patient permission.

Most writers contend that the ethics committee should act as a patient's advocate insofar as it is concerned with protecting the patient's interests, rather than interests of the hospital or of the treating team. It may be difficult to be a patient advocate without having access to confidential information, yet that does not answer the question: what justifies the ethics committee's gaining access to personal information about patients? If the committee wishes to act as a patient advocate, it could ask permission from patients to do so. It is not obvious that the committee as advocate is in the same position as a medical consultant. To the limited extent that the committee is involved in treatment decisions, can the committee be construed as a member of the treatment team?

Disclosures of private information to ethics committees cannot be justified merely because the disclosures will benefit the patient. If the disclosures are not otherwise covered within the bounds of the doctor-patient relationship or are not required by law, then disclosures to the ethics committee should not be made unless the patient gives prior consent. If legal regulation requires that ethics committees review specific treatment decisions, then the problem of patient consent changes, but the problem of *notice* (that is, notifying the patient that information is to be released to the committee) remains. If review (and thus disclosure) were legally required, the situation would parallel other previously noted reporting requirements.

Substantial disagreement exists about whether or not the patient (that is, either the patient or the person who is authorized to give consent for the patient) must be notified whenever disclosures are made to ethics committees. Most of the few writers who have written on this topic advocate that patients always be notified when an ethics committee reviews their case, and some state that patients must be asked for permission. There are a number of problems both with giving notice and with requesting consent (see, especially, pp. 58–61). It is an area of uncertainty and committees would be advised to consider the matter carefully before reviewing cases without patient permission or notice.

It is our belief that, in order to honor patient's claims to confidentiality and to demonstrate appropriate respect for patients, notice should be given to patients whenever their case is reviewed by the committee or by a subgroup of the committee. Should there be a decision not to notify the patient, members should be very clear about why they have decided to take this path. This might occur, for example, when there is a disagreement between physician and nurse about how much information should be given to the patient. Informing the patient of the dispute makes the resolution much more difficult. Furthermore, physicians may be unwilling to come to the committee if they have to inform their patients of the consultation. This is a very difficult issue and ethics committees will need to grapple seriously with it. The commitment to patient autonomy sharply conflicts with professional beneficence in this situation.

Another problem that ethics committees must consider with respect to the obligations of confidentiality is whether or not the presence of lay members on the committee affects the way in which the patient's claim to confidentiality or to notice of disclosure can be perceived. Arguably, the presence of lay members on the committee decreases the committee's claim to be like a member of the treatment team itself or a medical consultant and increases the need to receive consent for disclosure to the committee or to give notice to the patient that disclosure is to be made.

A final problem for the committee members is that of redisclosure. The cases that come to the ethics committee are likely to be extraordinarily complex but of significant educational value to ethics committee members at other hospitals, of great interest to the media, and of importance to public understanding of the dilemmas created by medical technology. If cases go to the courts, most claims to confidentiality are lost and, not infrequently, the medical record itself becomes part of the public record. When cases do not become a matter of public record and when no disclosure is legally required, ethics committees have an obligation to honor the patient's expectation of confidentiality. If the committee believes that the information should be redisclosed, then it should ask the patient for specific permission.

Inevitably, particularly interesting cases will be discussed in conference circuits and institutional "grapevines." When they are the subject at educational meetings, committee members should be very careful to protect the patient's identity and usually should alter aspects of the case to preclude the possibility of patient identification. The value of these cases as an educational instrument may be diminished somewhat by altering significant facts, but the patient's claims to confidentiality are of greater moral weight than the possible educational value, unless the patient has specifically authorized the redisclosure.

When controversial cases arise, the media frequently learn of them. If the ethics committee has been consulted about the case, the press is likely to seek information from the chairman or from individual members. The press holds the public's right to know as its highest value, but the ethics committee does not have to accept that priority. In the absence of patient consent or legal requirement, the ethics committee members have no moral or legal right to disclose any information about the case to anyone outside the hospital. The situation can be very problematic when the patient is a child or is otherwise incompetent and the problem derives from potential conflicts between the interests of the patient and the interests of the surrogate decision maker, be it parent, family member, or legal guardian. The committee should be very careful to try to sharply distinguish between disclosures that serve the interests of the hospital, disclosures that serve the interests of the patient, and disclosures that serve the interests of the press. The committee should, in these instances, serve the interest of the patient which, in the absence of patient consent, is to preserve the confidentiality of information the committee has about the patient. If the interests of the hospital need to be served, then it is the hospital itself that should undertake such disclosures, not the committee members.

In this Andy Warhol world in which everyone gets to be famous for 15 minutes, the attention of the media can be very seductive. To protect patients, ethics committees might want to consider adopting a standard policy of "no comment" to all public requests for information about specific cases. All inquiries about specific cases should be routed to the hospital administration, which usually has someone responsible for public relations. This is an area where dragons are rife. In a controversial case the demand for information is high, and it is easy but not always wise to conclude that it is better to accede to the demand rather than to permit erroneous information to be used. Furthermore, ethics committees were established in part to make sure that there would be public accountability. Nevertheless, it is probably better not to try to provide either accuracy or accountability through a 30-second news bite. If information is to be provided by the ethics committee, the patient's permission must be sought and the release of information should be coordinated with the hospital administration. This prohibition should not be interpreted generally, however. Ethics committees can and perhaps should provide *general* information to the media as a means of public education about ethical issues in health care.

In addition to news writers, feature writers may also be interested in exploring the committee's work. Here, the concern is not with a specific "hot" case, but with representative cases. The attention from the press may be flattering and members may not think unkindly about seeing themselves on the evening news or reading about themselves in the Sunday paper. Although they may start out discussing general issues, they will have a strong tendency to begin reminiscing about "one case in which a baby's parents—both of them were still teenagers working at a local McDonald's—didn't want to consent to surgery for their child with Down's syndrome and a duodenal atresia. The ethics committee, the doctors, and the parents—we all got the situation straightened out and that baby is now a joy to her parents." This may be good publicity for the ethics committee and the hospital and the bioethics movement, but it violates the committee's duty of confidentiality to the parents. It may not seem as if the family has been identified, but specifying the parents' ages and employment, which gives the story an appealing specificity, clearly breaches the family's claim to confidentiality. If specific cases with identifying facts are to be discussed with news people, then the patient and family must first give their consent to the disclosure.

Many people justify using this kind of detail because it explains the context of the situation more fully and thus explains the problem more effectively (the parents were young, unskilled, and had little money) and because there is very little real risk of anyone identifying the family or, if they did, of any harm coming from it. After all, no one is saying anything bad or critical about them. A duty of confidentiality, however, does not include permission to make decisions based upon judgment of the degree of risk or of harm to the patient. If specific cases are to be publicly discussed, no identifying characteristics should be included without permission. A rule of thumb might be: if the family members heard or read the case, would they realize that it referred to them? If they would, the statements should not be made. To use these cases may require altering details. If the case cannot be used effectively when details are changed to protect the patient and family, then the case should not be used.

Many of the cases that come before ethics committees are useful as educational vehicles. Because medical education is frequently case-based, there is a natural tendency to use the particularly complex case as a basis of either a written article or a verbal presentation at conferences or lectures. Although the risk of identities being disclosed or of injury being done to the patient as a result of a case being used in this way is even more remote than in media presentations, we still urge that patient confidentiality be protected. If cases are not a matter of public record, details should be altered so there is no prospect that the patient would be identifiable to himself or herself, to family, or to friends.

Ethics Committees' Claims to Privilege and Confidentiality

The claim is frequently made that the ethics committee should be entitled to claim complete confidentiality for its actions, just as a medical review committee is legally protected from discoverability. However, it is important not to confuse understandable desires for immunity and nondiscoverability with legitimate claims to confidentiality. Immunity and nondiscoverability refer to privilege, to legal protections that could be statutorily provided for the ethics committee's deliberations as a matter of public policy. A committee's claim to privilege for its own records will depend upon the particular state's laws and court decisions.

Whether the committee itself has a moral claim to confidentiality is another matter. That claim will depend upon whether or not it appears that there is a legitimate claim to a right of privacy that has been given up to receive some benefit. It does not appear that any member of the committee could make such a claim. Committee membership is voluntary, presumably, and any private information that is divulged by members would also appear to be voluntary. It is also not clear what information would be divulged in the course of committee work that would leave the members potentially vulnerable or stigmatized. It does not appear that, in ordinary circumstances, committee members themselves have any legitimate claim on one another to confidentiality. Although ordinary rules of human behavior would demand that members behave discreetly with respect to disclosing comments made by other committee members in the course of committee deliberations, a strict

claim to confidentiality could not be routinely claimed.

Nonmembers who may appear before the committee may be able to make such a claim much more easily. For example, should members of the treatment team be asked, expected, or required to confer with the committee, they have a legitimate claim to confidentiality, the more so if their presence is required, either officially or unofficially. Similarly, if family members were to confer with the committee, any information they provided should be held as confidential, because the committee has a potentially coercive role with respect to acquiring information.

There is not now any specific legal protection for persons (including physicians, nurses, social workers, chaplains, or family members) who provide information to the committee. In the absence of clear legal protections, committees have a distinct moral obligation to notify nonmembers who provide them with "personal" information *either* that it does not regard this as private information carrying an obligation of confidentiality *or* that it considers the information confidential and will not disclose it beyond the committee unless legally ordered to do so. This notice could be very difficult, for example, in a case involving treatment of a handicapped newborn in which the committee might assume an obligation to report the parents for child abuse, on the basis of information that the parents have provided. The parents should be informed prior to their discussing the matter with the committee how their information may be used and to whom it may be revealed.

If committees wish to maximize their offer of confidentiality to nonmembers, then they should consider how they might keep records that do not put these people at undue and inappropriate risk should there be a requirement that the records be disclosed. The committee needs to be able openly to explain its own actions at the same time that it shields information that patients and other nonmembers have provided. There may be times when these goals cannot both be attained. However, the committee should avoid breaching obligations of confidentiality. Making an unauthorized disclosure of confidential information is a very serious matter and should not be done hastily nor taken lightly. Gaining consent for voluntary disclosures and giving notice for legally required disclosures are better methods of achieving the same end.

References

Bruce, J. A. C. *Privacy and Confidentiality of Health Care Information.* Chicago: American Hospital Publishing, Inc. 1984, pp. 27-70.

Cranford, R. E., Hester, F. A., and Ashley, B. Z. Institutional ethics committees: Issues of confidentiality and immunity. *Law, Med Health Care.* 1985. 13(2):52-60.

Fost, N., and Cohen, S. Ethical issues regarding case reports: To publish or perish the thought. *Clin Research.* 1977. 24(4):269-73.

Harard, J. Medical confidence. *J Med Ethics.* 1985. 11:8-11.

Winslade, W. J. Privacy and confidentiality in medical records. *J Legal Med.* 1981. 3(4):497-533.

Chapter **12**

Treatment Decision Making

Competence and Consent

Both the law and the ethical principle of respect for persons and individual autonomy require that adult patients either consent to or refuse recommended treatment. In order for the consent or refusal to be valid, the patient must be competent. *Competency* is a legal term and is specific to a situation or to a task. It is not defined in general terms, but with respect to whether an individual is or is not competent to do some actual task. For example, one might be competent to make a will but not competent to handle money. Court determinations of competency customarily focus on whether the person understands the purpose, meaning, and implications of a specific activity and is able to make reasoned decisions based upon that knowledge. Much has been written about competency but there is very little consensus about how to handle competency questions in the health care setting.

Adults (however the term is defined by the state) are presumed to be competent. A *determination* of incompetency must be made by a court. Physicians, however, are frequently expected to *assess* competency and, should a court hearing be necessary, they will probably be expected to provide testimony about their assessment. Psychiatrists are often asked to help in assessing the presence of conditions that might impair the patient's ability to understand information and to make reasoned decisions. The comatose patient clearly lacks competence in every cognitive dimension. For most patients, however, matters are less clear. Competence can be impaired but not absent; it can be transitory; it can be spotty, that is, impaired only in specific matters. A patient might be cognitively competent regarding all but one topic and thus might not

be competent to make a particular medical decision, although one could conclude that the patient was competent to make medical decisions generally.

As a matter of fact (if not of ethics), little concern is paid to competency so long as the patient follows the physician's recommendations. Questions of competency arise most frequently when the patient wishes to pursue a course of action that the physician or the family does not endorse. Unfortunately, this leads to a very paternalistic manner of handling competency and consent. To counter this paternalistic tendency, many writers have urged that competency and consent be handled more formally in order to ensure that respect for persons and for patient autonomy is properly addressed.

Accepting consent from incompetent patients does not demonstrate respect either for persons or for patient autonomy. When a patient lacks competency, it is argued, someone should act in the patient's stead and ensure that his or her interests and wishes, if known, are honored. Although this is ethically appropriate, it may be practically cumbersome if the surrogate needs legal authority to consent, especially when consent is sought for very minor forms of treatment. In response to this pragmatic problem, several writers have suggested methods that balance respect for patient autonomy with the physician's beneficent duty to protect the patient's well-being.[1] These methods may address the moral issues, but may not respond to the legal demands unique to each state.

In one such scheme, stages of competence are defined by relating the stages to progressively higher levels of the complexity of the treatment decision that is to be made. Stage I competency applies to acute illness and requires that patients be aware and willing to assent to standard treatment or to refuse futile treatment. Only infants, very young children, and unconscious, severely retarded, or acutely psychotic patients do not rise to this standard. Stage II competency applies to chronic illness and to treatments with higher risks and less clear benefits. It requires the patient to be able to understand the information and to make a choice. To be considered competent, patients do not need to be able to explain their choices. Patients with severe mood disorders, memory loss, or dementia would not reach stage II competency, but mature adolescents, mildly retarded persons, and patients with some personality disorders ordinarily would. Stage III competency applies to refusal of standard life-saving treatment. It requires the patient to be able to appreciate the nature of the choice and to articulate some rational basis for it. Patients in a state of emotional shock, hysteria, or severe anxiety, for example, are unlikely to achieve this level of competence.

This schema is not unlike those devised by others, especially in the treatment of the mentally ill.[2] The general thrust of most writers on competence is that the greater the risk, the greater the degree of competence that should be required to make treatment decisions. This is true whether or not the physician recommends the particular treatment. When the risk is great and the probability of the risk is high, even more concern should be paid to the issue of competence.

Ethics committees that provide consultation may find themselves inquiring about the patient's competence, only to be told, "Yes, the patient is competent." Because competence is, for the most part, vaguely defined and because idiosyncratic meanings are quite common, committee members should be particularly concerned about the basis of this judgment of competence or incompetence. Some people believe that all mentally ill people are incompetent; some believe that all acutely ill people are under too much stress to be genuinely competent to make decisions; some believe that a patient's wishes should always be honored if he or she seems generally competent; and some believe that ambivalence implies incompetence.[3] The ethics committee needs to know the specific facts that led to the conclusion that the patient is incompetent to make the decisions that are being contemplated. There is a presumption of competency. If there are doubts about the patient's competence, then a court of law is the only place where a legal determination of incompetency can be made. Resorting to a legal determination is necessary only when there is uncertainty or disagreement about the patient's competence, when the patient voices any opposition to the treatment, or when the treatment is particularly risky.

When an adult patient has been determined legally incompetent, a conservator will be appointed. In some states, the person appointed by the courts is called a *conservator* if the person is an incompetent adult and a *guardian* if the person is a minor. The specific nature of the appointment will determine the scope of the conservator's authority. If the appointment has been sought in order to make medical decisions, then that will probably be included in the conservator's powers. In some cases, however, further application to the courts is required for specific kinds of medical decisions. In general, guardianship or conservatorship powers do not permit the conservator or guardian to give proxy consent for sterilization, abortion, electroconvulsive therapy (ECT, or shock treatment), or psychosurgery. Mental health conservatorships do not customarily include authority for consenting to any medical treatment other than treatment for the mental illness.

When a patient who is clearly incompetent (unconscious, for example) arrives at the hospital and needs immediate life-saving treatment, no consent is required. Emergency treatment does not require explicit consent because the patient is usually not able to express autonomous decisions and in cases of questionable competence there is insufficient time to determine incompetency. Consent is implied in emergency circumstances, whereas both urgent and elective treatment always require valid, explicit consent. Urgent treatment might be defined as that required in situations in which the patient's condition will deteriorate if he or she is not treated promptly, but death is not imminent or, perhaps, even probable.

Who makes decisions for incompetent patients? In many and perhaps most hospitals, family members (spouses, children, parents) routinely consent to treatment for adult incompetent patients. The strict legality of familial consent varies from state to state. In some states, there is no statutory authority for accepting familial consent for adult patients who have not been judged legally incompetent. There may, however, be judicial authority. As a practical matter, physicians and hospitals will probably continue to accept family consent in such situations so long as the family members and the physicians agree, even if there is no specific legal authority for doing so.

Under normal circumstances, parents are entitled to consent to or refuse treatment for their minor children. Under child-abuse-law definitions of medical neglect, they are also legally obligated to consent to necessary medical care for their minor children. The new Baby Doe laws (the 1984 amendments to the federal Child Abuse Prevention and Treatment Act) contain provisions for ensuring consent to treatment when parents refuse consent for seriously ill newborns whose lives can be prolonged, despite severe handicapping conditions. Should parents refuse to consent to medically necessary treatment for their seriously ill newborn, hospitals may go directly to the courts to request judicial consent or to the state child protective services agency, which will arrange to obtain consent. In either case, consent to treatment must be obtained before treatment is provided. There is an exception to this: the federal legislation requires that, if there is a disagreement about whether or not medical treatment is appropriate, all care necessary to keep the infant alive must be provided until the disagreement is resolved. At that time, if treatment is to be continued, appropriate consent is given.

Although parents must consent to or refuse treatment for adolescent minor children, ethical issues arise in the treatment of adolescents who are not considered to be competent as a matter of law, but who may have the capacities that are required to demonstrate competency in adults. They may be able to understand not only the nature of their situation but also the risks and benefits of accepting and refusing treatment, and they may be able to make reasoned judgments. However, their consent alone is not legally acceptable. Respect for their real competencies, however, means that they, too, should be asked to consent and that, when consent is lacking, an ethical problem is present. It should be noted that adolescent minors are entitled in many states to obtain birth control devices and drugs, abortions, and treatment for venereal disease, as well as to receive outpatient mental health care, without parental consent. Legally emancipated minors can consent to any treatment, as would any adult. Definitions of legal emancipation differ from state to state, but they customarily include such categories as being married, being financially independent, being a member of the armed forces, and so on.

When judicial approval is sought for treating children (usually in situations of conflict between family members or between the family and the physician), it is often available quickly and, in some states, often by telephone. The courts tend to defer to medical judgment in such cases. When there is a disagreement about the need for treatment of an adult patient, court processes will be much slower, even if the need is urgent (but not an emergency). Hospitals usually have considerable experience in obtaining consent to medical procedures for incompetent patients, especially those without families.

Frequently, cases are taken to the courts not because there is any real disagreement about whether treatment should be provided but because the hospitals or physicians do not wish to act in an uncertain area in the absence of judicial approval. They wish to avoid any litigation or risk of liability. In most states, the courts hearing such cases attempt to provide decisions that will provide guidance to other physicians in other hospitals within their jurisdiction so that every case need not be brought to the courts. In Massachusetts, the courts are more inclined to urge an active role for the judiciary in case-by-case decision making. In most other states, there is less interest in having the courts make these decisions. Several appellate court decisions have agreed that removing life-support systems from permanently unconscious patients is acceptable with family approval and without court involvement.

Advance Directives for Patients

In recent years, the public has become increasingly aware of medicine's new capabilities for keeping dying patients alive for extended periods of time. In addition, the public understands something about physicians' tendencies to use this technology, even when families (and patients, in some cases) do not wish further treatment to be pursued. From this awareness, the "right to die" claim has grown. This phrase does not represent a moral claim to a right to die. Rather, it is an expression of an *autonomy* claim; the patient is claiming a right to refuse treatment, even though the refusal may lead to his or her death. Forty states and the District of Columbia have either statutory or judicial authority for the patient's right to refuse life-prolonging treatment. In the other states, the law of informed consent presumably provides authority for the refusal of treatment.

Because patients are very likely to have become incompetent to express their preferences by the time they might want to refuse further treatment, the "living will" was developed. The original purpose of living wills was to provide a formal (though not official) method for persons to indicate their desire to refuse treatment under certain conditions. Living will documents typically contained such statements as, "If the time should come when I am no longer able to make decisions and my death is imminent, then I do not wish to receive heroic or extraordinary treatment." These documents had no legal standing: they were only advisory and were a means of ensuring that health care professionals were aware of a person's general preferences.

Because physicians did not always accept these documents as determinative, a movement began in the 1970s to provide legally authorized and legally binding documents that would require physicians to abide by a patient's wishes if the patient had signed the form recognized by the state. These statutes are sometimes referred to as "living will legislation," as "natural death acts," or as "directives to physicians."

During the 1980s, because the legislatively approved documents often applied in only a narrow range of circumstances, new attempts have been made to provide legal authority for foregoing treatment when patients are no longer competent to make their wishes known. This legislation is referred to as a "durable power of attorney statute."

These are the three forms of patient directives: nonlegally recognized living wills; statutorily-authorized living wills, directives to physicians, or natural death act directives; and durable powers of attorney that include authorization for health care decision making. Many writers refer to the natural death act directive as a form of living will, but there is considerable disagreement about this. For example, a writer may say that California recognizes living wills because it has a natural death act, whereas another writer may say that California does not recognize living wills but does recognize a natural death act directive because it has such a statute. In fact, the California natural death act specifically states that the directive to physicians is not a living will.

Any competent adult can sign any of these directives as a means of indicating his or her preferences. The document is *advisory only,* however, unless the individual resides in a state that has legally recognized such a document either judicially or, more commonly, legislatively.

Ethics committee members need to know the differences between these forms and the legal status of each in their own state. In general, a patient is better off signing a legally recognized directive rather than one that is only advisory, that is, one that a health care professional is not legally obliged to honor.

Nonlegislatively Authorized Living Wills

A living will is a personal expression of an individual's preference for the extent of medical treatment desired. It may, in some instances, also name a person to make decisions for the person should he or she become incompetent to do so. Living wills may be initiated, rewritten, or withdrawn by the individual at any time. Preprinted forms are available, such as the living wills prepared by the Concern for Dying and by the Society for the Right to Die, or the Christian Affirmation of Life statement prepared by the Catholic Hospital Association. There are other formulations of living wills, as well. People may choose to write

their own statements about the extent of treatment they want. When a state recognizes a living will only as a statement of an individual's preferences, then it may be written in any form. If a state statutorily recognizes a living will, it is likely to require a specific form.

When considering living wills, ethics committees need to be particularly concerned about their legal status: are they legally binding documents or are they merely informational and advisory? From the perspective of ethics committees, of course, these documents should carry considerable moral force.

Legislators have sometimes been reluctant to make living wills legally binding for a number of reasons. First, they are aware that a person's preferences might change during a medical crisis, but the patient might not be able to convey such a change of mind; moreover, health care professionals might not know how to interpret the statement of preference once the patient had become incompetent. Second, because patients have a moral right to life-saving or life-extending treatment, legislators question whether patients can give up that right in advance of the actual situation. Third, many believe that the documents must, of necessity, be worded generally in order to cover whatever medical crisis befalls the person, but that generality makes it difficult and sometimes impossible to know how to apply the directive "correctly" in the actual medical situation. Finally, there has been real fear that if such documents came to be widely used, the potential for abuse would be enormous. For example, aged or socially "unproductive" individuals might not receive treatment under the guise of honoring vague or even implied living will statements.

A person who prepares a living will should discuss his or her wishes with family members as well as with the primary physician. If a patient or a member of his or her family presents a living will to hospital personnel, it should be placed in the medical record according to hospital procedure.

Legislatively Authorized Living Wills and Natural Death Act Directives

Legislatively authorized living wills or natural death act directives vary from state to state, but they generally include the following:

- An acknowledgment of an adult's right to forego medical treatment in the event of a terminal condition
- Immunity from criminal and civil liability for the health care professionals who act in accordance with the patient directive

- A statement about the circumstances (usually a terminal illness) under which a directive is applied and, sometimes, a statement that death is imminent
- A statement about the kind of procedures that can be refused (for example, artificial procedures or procedures that only prolong the dying process)
- The form the directive must take
- Procedures for executing a directive, including requirements for witnesses or notarization
- Procedures for revoking a directive
- The period during which the directive is in effect
- The obligation of a physician who is unwilling to honor the terms of a directive to transfer the care of the patient to a physician who will do so

In addition, many statutes invalidate the directive when the patient is a pregnant woman; provide penalties for forging or intentionally destroying a patient's directive; state that the patient's currently expressed wishes supersede any wishes included in a directive; and state that the directive does not affect insurance or health benefits, nor does the patient's death when treatment is foregone constitute a suicide or mercy killing. Finally, a few states provide proxy appointments and procedures for decision making for incompetent patients who have not signed directives.[4]

The directive or a copy of the directive should be placed in the patient's medical record. Many institutions also place some kind of symbol on the front cover of the patient's record indicating that it contains a natural death act or other patient directive.

Durable Power of Attorney for Health Care

All states have durable power of attorney statutes. These documents do not customarily include specific language permitting the "attorney in fact" to consent to or to refuse medical care. (Pennsylvania and Colorado durable power of attorney statutes do specifically include authorization for medical care decision making.) Some writers have suggested that a standard durable power of attorney could include such language and hospitals and physicians would be obliged to honor it. Hospital attorneys, however, have been less inclined to accept this kind of authority for refusing life-prolonging treatment. (The New York State attorney general has issued an opinion stating that specific delegation of health care decision making would be acceptable in that state.)

As a result, some states have considered durable power of attorney for health care legislation. California was the first state to pass specific legislation of this sort. This legislation provides authority for the named attorney-in-fact to consent to or to refuse specific forms of life-prolonging care. The person signing the durable power may provide either general instructions or very precise instructions as to how he or she wishes the attorney-in-fact to exercise his or her decision-making power. Consent for some kinds of medical treatment may be statutorily denied. (For example, in California the attorney-in-fact cannot consent to electroconvulsive therapy, abortion, psychosurgery, or mental hospital commitment or treatment.) The durable power of attorney for health care is triggered whenever the "principal," the person signing the document, becomes incompetent, regardless of whether he or she is terminally ill or death is imminent.

The attorney-in-fact (the proxy or surrogate decision maker) has the same legal authority to give or withhold consent as the patient would have if competent (other than any statutorily stated exceptions). The proxy's responsibilities to make health care decisions include consent, refusal of consent, and withdrawal of consent to most care, treatment, service, or procedures. The proxy's decisions are also subject to any limitations or requirements that the individual has included in the document. The proxy must act consistently with the individual's desires, if they are known, and in the individual's best interests, if the desires are not specified.

Uniform Anatomical Gift Act

The Uniform Anatomical Gift Act permits persons to authorize the donation, at the time of death, of his or her body or body parts for organ transplantation, research, or education. Fifty states and the District of Columbia have adopted the Uniform Anatomical Gift Act. The individual may donate his or her body or its parts by will or by other document or card, signed by the individual. The document may be revoked orally (in the presence of two witnesses and communicated to the donee, or, when the individual has a terminal illness or injury, by telling the attending physician and communicating it to the donee); in writing; or by destroying the document (if it has not been delivered to a donee).

Notes

1. See, for example, Drane, J. F. Competency to give an informed consent. *JAMA*. 1984. 252(10)925-7; Drane, J.F. The many faces of competency. *Hastings Cent Rep*. 1985. 15(2):17-21.

2. The mentally ill are not, by definition, incompetent. Their level of competence must be assessed, just as with any other patient, although they usually can be treated for

their mental illness without giving consent if they meet state requirements for involuntary commitment or certification. In some states, however, they may not be treated for any medical conditions other than mental illness, without legally given consent.

3. Patients who are choosing to forego life-sustaining treatment almost always show some ambivalence. For an example of one court's handling of the relationship between competence and ambivalence, see *Bartling v. Superior Court,* p.276.

4. For further discussion of these points, see Society for the Right to Die. *The Physician and the Hopelessly Ill Patient.* New York: Society for the Right to Die, 1985, p. 39.

References

American Hospital Association, Special Committee on Biomedical Ethics. *Values in Conflict: Resolving Ethical Issues in Hospital Care.* Chicago: AHA, 1985, pp. 67-74.

California Medical Association. *Your Health Care: Who Will Decide When You Can't?* Durable Power of Attorney for Health Care: Patient Guidelines. San Francisco, CA: CMA, 1984.

Collin, F. J., and Meyers, D. W. Using a durable power of attorney for the authorization of withdrawal of medical care. *Estate Planning.* Sept. 1984. 282-7.

Culver, C. M., and Gert, B. Basic ethical concepts in neurological practice. *Seminars Neurol.* 1984. 4(1):1-8.

Michel, V. Competence to make medical decisions. *Ethical Currents.* 1985. 5:6.

President's Commission for the Study of Ethical Problems in Medicine and Biomedical and Behavioral Research. *Deciding to Forego Treatment.* Appendix D, Natural death statutes and proposals; Appendix E, Statutes and proposals to empower appointment of proxies. Washington, DC: U.S. Government Printing Office, 1983, pp. 391-438.

Roth, L. R., Meisel, A., and Lidz, C. W. Tests of competency to consent to treatment. *Am J Psychiatry.* 1977. 134:3.

Society for the Right to Die. *The physician and the hopelessly ill patient.* New York: Society for the Right to Die, 1985.

Chapter 13

Committee Liability

Because ethics committees are so new, there has been no litigation that would provide us with a clear sense of how the courts will look at the actions of the committees with respect to criminal and civil liability. This section is not intended to give legal advice but rather to sensitize committee members to the issues involved in legal liability and to help them to avoid situations wherein they might find themselves, as a group or as individuals, held liable for their actions. It is not possible, of course, to act in such a way as to avoid all possibility of someone's filing a suit against the committee or its members. Anyone may sue. If a committee conducts its actions conscientiously and sensitively, however, there is little likelihood of any finding of liability.

The risk of liability is directly related to the role the committee plays in the hospital. When the committee is given or takes a decision-making role, there is much greater risk of liability. This is not the primary reason that committees should function only in an advisory capacity with respect to specific cases. It is, however, a subsidiary reason. Even if the committee's role is such that it has very little risk of legal liability, the hospital should make certain that all members are appropriately insured against liability risks. It may be that all members of a committee are covered under existing hospital policies. However, any lay members or other members who are not hospital employees or staff physicians may not be automatically insured. Specific action must be taken to protect any members not covered. Nonhospital employees who are being asked to contribute time and expertise to the committee's work should not be expected to finance their own defense in case a legal suit is filed.

Some writers have urged that nonhospital ethics committee members be given written statements by the hospital with respect to this insurance coverage. In addition, some have suggested that the hospital provide insurance indemnification for any judgment that exceeds the policy limits. Although this question of protecting members from the costs of legal suits is often discussed, it is our impression that seldom is there any follow-up by the hospital administration. The risk of suit is probably small; the risk of liability is even smaller. Yet, if the committee waits until a suit is filed to determine how the hospital will protect them, it will be of little matter that the risk was small.

Criminal Liability

There is very little likelihood that a committee would be either charged with or found criminally liable for any of its actions. Physicians are much closer to the actual decisions, and they are rarely charged with any kind of criminal action. (See, for example, the case of *Barber* v. *Superior Court,* chapter 14, in which Doctors Barber and Nejdl were criminally charged in the death of Clarence Herbert. The court rejected the contention that there was a potential for criminal liability in such a situation and dismissed the case.)

Criminal liability requires that there be reason to believe that the person or persons charged have violated some kind of law. This may involve either performing an act or failing to perform an act that the person or persons have a duty to perform. If an ethics committee had a statutory obligation to protect patients but failed to do so, then they might be criminally charged. Ethics committees have no such duty nor any other duty, to the best of our judgment, that would place them at risk for any kind of criminal liability. Where there is a duty to report child abuse, failure to do so is a crime in most states. The 1984 amendments to the Child Abuse Protection and Treatment Act anticipate that medical neglect of infants will be included as an instance of child abuse under state laws. States' actions in this area may, therefore, create a potential for criminal liability for ethics committee members. Committees will need to assess carefully their own state's position on this matter.

Civil Liability

Civil liability—tort liability—involves four elements. For a person or a group to be found civilly liable for a tort (that is, a *wrong* or *wrongful act*), four elements must be met and proved. First, the individual (or group) must have a duty. Second, he or she must breach that duty. Third, there must be an injury. And, fourth, the injury must be caused by the breach of duty. Three kinds of tort might be of concern to ethics committee members: negligence, intentional harm to a patient, and invasion of privacy.

A court might find a committee or its members guilty of *negligence* if the committee made recommendations that were decisive or that they knew would be strongly relied upon for a decision and if the recommendations resulted from improper or poorly thought out procedures, or from erroneous or insufficient information. Committees that provide only advisory opinions cannot always know how influential their advice may be. They can, however, design thorough procedures for acquiring information and for ensuring adequate consideration of all factors before making recommendations. A committee should not, for example, depend upon one person only for the information about a case. Different people interpret events in different ways. Unless the committee has an opportunity to hear from all or, at least, many of the people involved, it will have no way of knowing whether it has gathered sufficient information about the facts and about the values at issue.

A charge of *intentional harm to the patient* might result from one or more committee members having a conflict of interest with regard to a recommendation on a specific case. For example, suppose the committee were asked to review prospectively the case of a patient whose cost of treatment would not be reimbursed. The issue is whether or not treatment should be terminated for ethical reasons. Some members of the committee may have a direct financial stake in the hospital's operations or their employment may be directly affected by such financial considerations. As a result, they may have a conflict of interest. The committee should carefully consider whether those members should participate in discussions or recommendations about the case. This consideration is especially important whenever the person with the conflict of interest is a particularly powerful or influential member of the committee, a hospital administrator or a hospital attorney, or a physician who has a proprietary interest in the hospital's finances. In the *Barber* case, it should be recalled, there was some talk that the decision to stop treatment was at least partially motivated by financial considerations, in that the hospital was a health maintenance organization.

Ethics committees have a duty to protect patient confidentiality. Thus, if they breach that duty and thereby cause harm to the patient, they may be found liable for *invasion of privacy*. Although confidentiality is a value with an extraordinarily long tradition in medicine, it is often treated casually in the hospital setting. Ethics committee members need to be very careful about protecting patient privacy. (For further discussion of confidentiality, see chapter 11.) Liability for the invasion of privacy of persons other than the patient is not so clear. Health care providers and family members who give information to the committee could conceivably be injured if the information they provide were not protected by committee members. For example, a nurse who provided information about a case might lose her job or the trust of her colleagues if the committee revealed the source of the information. The question of confidentiality for those who give information to ethics committees in the course of case reviews is a very thorny one. If the committee promises confidentiality to these individuals, then it clearly has a duty to provide it. If the duty is breached and an injury is thereby caused, liability could follow.

Committee Immunity from Discoverability

If the eithics committee is constituted as a medical staff committee, its minutes and records of deliberation may be nondiscoverable. For more discussion of this issue, see "Organizational Placement" in chapter 5 and "Privacy, Confidentiality, and Privilege" in chapter 11.

Potential Problems with Respect to Committee Liability

The general purpose of an ethics committee is to ensure that adequate consideration is given to the ethical dimensions of clinical care. In the course of their activities, members may become aware of ethical, legal, or medical improprieties. The question of what to do with this information may be very problematic. In fact, the committee structure itself may exacerbate the problem by its tendency to diffuse a sense of personal responsibility. For example, although a person acting in his or her independent capacity would have unhesitatingly discussed and pursued a questionable situation with a superior, he or she as a committee member might feel absolved of further responsibility, having turned the issue over to the committee, even if the committee does nothing about it. Committees as groups often find themselves operating within very limited mandates or with a tenuous political position. As a result, they may be reluctant to pursue certain issues for fear of endangering their very existence. Such muddy situations, in which responsibilities and lines of authority are unclear, create a real potential for actions that can breed lawsuits.

Overall, the presence of ethics committees should reduce exposure to litigation rather than increase it. Being a member of an ethics committee does not appear to be a very risky matter with respect to legal liability. Because important values are at issue, however, the potential for liability can increase if the committee and its members do not take their responsibilities seriously and thoughtfully. A committee that begins to review cases at its first meeting is taking much greater risks than a committee that first makes sure that its members have received some specific education about the committee's roles and responsibilities, as well as the nature of biomedical ethics and ethical analysis, before undertaking a review function.

Currently no standard of conduct for ethics committees is universally accepted. A finding of liability would require that the committee is not meeting *some* standard. Even though that standard does not exist in law today, it would be entirely possible for a judge or jury to conclude that specific practices were simply inadequate and that any reasonable person would find them so. As reasonable people, ethics committee members should learn to look critically at their own practices. They should ask what would happen if their actions and procedures were described objectively to patients, their families, or to the general public. Would they appear to be acting responsibly? If so, they probably have little reason to fear liability.

Reference

Hirsch, H. Interview: Establish ethics committees to minimize liability, authority advises. *Hosp Risk Manage.* 1981. 3(4):45-8.

Chapter 14

Landmark Cases

This chapter includes summaries of a number of important court decisions in the area of bioethics. The decisions in these cases are frequently referred to in the bioethics literature, in which it is often assumed that the reader is familiar with the facts of the cases as well as the import of the decisions. Because copies of court decisions are not always easy to procure without easy access to a law library, these summaries are included to help ethics committee members become familiar with relevant cases. (Citations are provided so that copies of the decisions can be obtained.) They are "landmark cases" in the sense that most are pivotal to the legal assessment of a specific issue. For example, the *Quinlan* decision was the first to address the issue of withdrawing ventilator support from a permanently unconscious patient and its reasoning was subsequently cited in many other cases involving the foregoing of life-sustaining treatment. The cases are arranged alphabetically by topic and chronologically within each topic.

Abortion

Roe v. Wade (410 U.S. 113, 1973)

This landmark decision overturned anti-abortion laws throughout the United States. The court based its decision on the right of privacy, but maintained that abortion is essentially a medical decision and is thus to be made by the physician in consultation with his or her patient. The court balanced the woman's interest in deciding to bear a child with the state's interests in protecting her health and in protecting fetal life. The fetus is found to be a potential person but not, under the constitution, a person. The decision provides a legislative-like schema that prohibits the states from passing legislation that will restrict a woman's access to abortion during either the first or second trimester, except that regulation of second trimester abortions is permissible if the intention is to protect the woman's health. States may, *if they choose,* prohibit all abortions after the fetus becomes viable (viability is a medical decision) except those intended to safeguard the woman's life and health.

Subsequent cases have established that although the woman can be required to give informed consent to the procedure, states cannot require spousal consent or, in the case of minors, parental consent unless they also provide an alternative judicial forum to review minors' decisions. States may, however, require parental notice in the case of minors requesting abortion. The Court has also made clear in various decisions that viability is a medical concept and is to be defined by medical practice, not by legislation.

With respect to funding, a series of decisions have held that neither city, county, state, nor federal government has any obligation to provide abortion funding to those who may otherwise be dependent upon public services or medical welfare. These funding decisions clearly establish that the right to abortion is, in a philosophical sense, a negative rather than a positive right. That is, the state may not interfere with a woman's access to abortion but has no duty to provide her with an abortion.

Roe v. Wade has been widely criticized by both the legal and the academic communities as a legal decision (separate from its content). The most recent U.S. Supreme Court decision involving abortion (*City of Akron v. Akron Center for Reproductive Health,* 1983) includes a dissent by Justice Sandra Day O'Connor that carefully analyzes one of the major problems with the decision, that is, the use of "medical viability" as the critical time period upon which hangs the state's ability to regulate abortion. Technological change is likely to move the date of viability ever earlier in pregnancy, creating conflicts with the second trimester rights established by *Roe*. At least in theory, viability as defined by the court could eventually be identical with conception. Even now, some writers argue that embryo transfer establishes a "window" of viability prior to implantation.

The decision is frequently thought to prohibit third trimester abortion and to grant a right to abortion on demand. Neither of these interpretations is accurate although, in practice, abortion on request is available because physicians have not chosen to involve themselves in any significant manner in the abortion decision; and third trimester abortions are performed very infrequently because physicians do not choose to perform them. (Many doctors, of course, would argue that there is no such thing as a third trimester abortion since in that stage it would be induced labor. However, if the intention in such procedures is to ensure that the fetus is not live-born, then this, too, should be characterized, for legal purposes, as an abortion.) Many states have passed legislation requiring that fetuses who are live-born in the course of an abortion receive the same medical care as would any other newborn infant. Some states have required a second physician to be present any time an abortion may result in a live birth.

Foregoing Treatment: Incompetent Patients

In the Matter of Karen Quinlan (70 NJ 10, 1976)

Karen Quinlan was unconscious, perhaps as a result of ingesting alcohol and barbiturates, when she arrived at the hospital. Her doctors believed that there was no probability that she would ever regain consciousness. Her father took this case to court, asking that he be named her guardian and be permitted to consent to discontinuing ventilatory support. Her physicians had refused to do this when the family had asked them. The New Jersey Attorney General and the County Prosecutor had both advised that turning off the respirator on a patient like Ms. Quinlan constituted criminal homicide. Several physicians testified that under current "medical standards, practice, and ethics," the respirator must be continued as long as the patient was not brain dead. The New Jersey

Supreme Court decided that the decision was not strictly medical and thus current medical standards need not be determinative. Mr. Quinlan had asserted his daughter's right of privacy as the justification for the request to terminate life support and the court accepted the relevance of this right both to the treatment termination decision and to Mr. Quinlan's right to assert the privacy right on his daughter's behalf. By connecting the treatment decision to the privacy right, the court eliminated the issue of criminal homicide.

Despite the court's acknowledgment of the importance and direct relevance of the privacy right, it did not ultimately permit that right as the sole basis for a decision to terminate treatment. Instead, the court judged that if an "ethics committee" (it meant, in fact, a *prognosis* committee) agreed with Quinlan's physician that there was "no reasonable possibility of Karen's ever emerging from her present comatose condition to a cognitive, sapient state," then, if the family and Ms. Quinlan's guardian agreed, the respirator could be withdrawn. (Although everyone had expected Quinlan to die when the respirator was withdrawn, she was successfully weaned from it and lived until June, 1985.)

Quinlan is significant because it was the first case to deal specifically with the question of withdrawing ventilatory support from a permanently unconscious patient. It is often cited as a source for the importance of the privacy right in these life-and-death decisions. As a result of the *Quinlan* case, many hospitals in New Jersey, where the decision is binding, formed ethics committees. Relatively fewer hospitals in other states formed such committees. These ethics committees, however, were not usually formed to deal only with prognosis confirmation (which the *Quinlan* court had specified as the committee's function).

Superintendent of Belchertown State School v. Saikewicz (370 NE2d 417, 1977)

Joseph Saikewicz was a 67-year-old profoundly retarded man with an IQ of 10 who had been institutionalized for 53 years. In 1976, he was found to be suffering from leukemia. Chemotherapy, the standard treatment, had a 30 percent to 50 percent probability of producing a remission of 2 to 13 months. The guardian *ad litem* (that is, a guardian appointed by the court for a single purpose; in this case, to determine whether Saikewicz should receive chemotherapy) recommended that chemotherapy *not* be given because it was less successful in older patients and because the side effects were painful and debilitating and because Saikewicz could not understand or cooperate with the treatment. The probate judge weighed the burdens and the benefits and noted that Saikewicz's quality of life, even if remission were achieved, was insufficient to justify treatment. The appellate court reviewed the lower decision and concluded that it was, in essence, correct, although the appellate court stressed that Saikewicz's quality of life could not be taken into consideration insofar as that referred to the fact that he was a profoundly retarded, institutionalized patient. That is, he could not be denied treatment on the basis of his handicaps. The decision also acknowledged the right of privacy as a right of personal determination. The court pointed out that incompetent patients should not be denied a right to refuse treatment. The appropriate standard for the decision maker was *substituted judgment*; that is, that which the incompetent patient would decide for himself or herself, "taking into account the present and future incompetency of the individual." Saikewicz died of pneumonia before the appellate court's written decision was published.

The *Saikewicz* decisions were widely criticized among the medical community because, unlike the *Quinlan* decision, they claimed that the courts were the appropriate decision makers in such cases. Furthermore, the decisions rejected the *Quinlan* endorsement of ethics committees. Massachusetts justices have continued to encourage judicial decision making or approval in problematic medical-ethical cases, but other states have not generally followed their lead.

The decision's primary importance lies in its attempt to extend autonomy to those who are incapable of exercising it. The appellate decision emphasizes the fact that even though most people choose chemotherapy when leukemia is diagnosed, it is possible that a particular competent individual, given his or her specific situation, might decide that the probable burdens of chemotherapy exceeded its possible benefits. Since the law would not force the average person's choices upon that person, then neither should it force them upon the incompetent patient simply because he or she is incapable of decision making. In order to give the incompetent patient access to "autonomous" choice, a proxy decision maker (in this case, the guardian *ad litem*, with the court's approval) is to make a substituted judgment, based upon the patient's previously expressed statements, values, and attitudes. If, as in the case of Joseph Saikewicz, nothing is known about what the patient would want, then the proxy is to cast himself imaginatively into the patient's role, trying to imagine what he or she would want if he or she could.

This distinction between a substituted judgment standard and a *best interests* standard is an important one in proxy decision making. Unfortunately, the court's opinion confuses the distinction somewhat by describing substituted judgment as a determination of the individual patient's "best interests." Ordinarily, a best interests standard means doing whatever most people would do for themselves or for their children in the same situation, that is, a reasonable person standard. As well, the "best interests" standard should take into account any unique characteristics of the individual for whom the decision is being made. In other words, the decision should be made to fit the specific person's best interests if there is reason to believe that they would differ from those of the ordinary person. Furthermore, the *Saikewicz* decision has been criticized on the grounds that a substituted judgment is impossible when the proxy has no authentic information about the incompetent patient's values, attitudes, and perspectives. In such a case, these critics argue, the proxy must choose whatever a reasonable person would choose since the proxy has no basis for a substituted judgment.

In the Matter of Shirley Dinnerstein (380 NE 2d 134, 1978)

Dinnerstein was a 67-year-old Alzheimer's syndrome patient in a vegetative state with serious coronary artery disease and uncontrollable high blood pressure. Her family and physician requested the court's permission to enter a "no-code" or do-not-resuscitate (DNR) order on the patient's chart. Their decision to request permission stemmed from *Saikewicz,* which suggested that all decisions to withhold or withdraw life-prolonging treatment from an incompetent patient must be approved by a court.

The appellate court distinguished the case from *Saikewicz* in that, in *Saikewicz,* treatment included the possibility of a return to the patient's normal life, whereas cardiopulmonary resuscitation (CPR) for Dinnerstein would not restore her condition to what it had normally been. Where the treatment might cure or significantly ameliorate the patient's condition, then a decision not to treat an incompetent patient required court approval. When treatment pertained to decisions about "what measures are appropriate to ease the imminent passing of an irreversibly, terminally ill patient," then the question depends upon medical competence, and should be made in light of the patient's "condition and history" and the family's wishes.

The *Dinnerstein* case articulates a widely held belief about the nature of DNR decisions. This court decision, moreover, appears to place DNR orders on the same footing as respirator withdrawal in the case of permanently unconscious patients. Thus, *Dinnerstein* is much closer to cases like *Quinlan* and *Eichner* (see the next discussion) than it is to *Saikewicz*.

Eichner v. Dillon (426 NY2d 517, 1980)

Brother Fox was 83 years old at the time he suffered cardiac arrest during a hernia operation. Although physicians were able to restore heart function, Brother Fox became permanently unconscious. Reverend Eichner, a close friend and religious superior, petitioned the court to authorize termination of respirator care. Several people testified as to Brother Fox's specific wishes *not* to be kept alive if he should become permanently comatose.

The court concluded that Brother Fox's "right to bodily self-determination" and right to privacy were not lost because he was incompetent, but contended that these rights needed to be weighed against the state's interests in preserving life, in protecting third parties, in maintaining the ethical integrity of the medical profession, and in preventing suicide. (These four state interests are always cited in cases involving the foregoing of treatment.) Finding that the state's interests were not compelling in this instance, the court established a procedure by which life-sustaining measures could be withdrawn. Like the *Quinlan* court, the *Fox* court required concurrence by a three-physician prognosis committee. When such agreement was given, then a legally authorized guardian might request withdrawal of treatment, a request that could be challenged by the attorney general, the district attorney, or a court-appointed guardian *ad litem*. The ultimate decision was to be made by the court. Although the court endorsed Fox's privacy rights and rights of bodily self-determination, its decision in this case does not clearly make the final decision about treatment withdrawal dependent upon the patient's having made his attitude or wishes known.

This case is important because it fits into the line of cases involving incompetent patients: like Saikewicz and Quinlan, Fox was incompetent. Unlike Saikewicz, Fox had not always been incompetent and unlike Quinlan, Fox had made clear and specific statements about his preferences in such a situation. The courts have moved carefully throughout the past few years in an attempt to draw very careful lines in deciding when treatment can be foregone.

Barber v. Superior Court (147 Cal.App.3d 1006, 1983)

Doctors Nejdl and Barber were charged with murder and conspiracy to commit murder following the death of Clarence Herbert, a patient under their care. Herbert went into cardiac arrest following routine surgery. He was resuscitated and placed on a respirator. After three days, the doctors concluded that Herbert would not recover consciousness, and his family consented to removal of the respirator. Herbert continued to breathe without the ventilator and, after two more days and with family consent, the patient's intravenous lines, providing food and fluids, were removed. The patient died several days later.

Prior to trial, the California Second District Appellate Court dismissed the charges against the doctors on the grounds that physicians have no duty to provide treatment that is ineffective. In the case of a permanently unconscious patient like Herbert, the court stated that decisions should be based on whether the treatment is proportionate or disproportionate; that is, whether the potential benefits outweigh the expected burdens. The decision suggests that when there is *no* possibility of a "return to cognitive and sapient life," then treatment benefits are so minimal that *any* burden would reasonably outweigh them. Thus, continuing life-support measures that had no prospect of returning Herbert to "cognitive and sapient life" was reasonably judged to be ineffective and not a part of the physicians' duty. Finally, the court found that, in the absence of legislation to the contrary, family members are appropriate surrogate decision makers even if they are not legal guardians.

Barber is an important case, first, because it involves criminal charges. Many writers have stated that the likelihood of criminal prosecution in medical cases involving bioethics is essentially nonexistent, but clearly the risk does exist. Beyond that, the decision is important because it establishes that the state does not always demand the preservation of biological life, that family members may consent to or refuse treatment for an incompetent patient, and that "medical" feeding (that is, technological means of providing food and fluids), at least in these circumstances, is a form of treatment, not a basic requirement of patient care.

The decision should be read narrowly on these last two issues, however. With respect to family consent, the court notes that Mrs. Herbert was the appropriate surrogate decision maker and that a court would have so concluded had it been consulted. Second, although the food and fluids statement is clear enough, the issue is so controversial that, in slightly different circumstances, a different conclusion might easily be drawn about the necessity of providing nutrition and hydration. By comparison, it should be noted that, in the Baby Doe legislation, "appropriate nutrition, hydration, and medication" are required even in those cases in which life-extending treatment is being withheld or withdrawn.

In the Matter of Claire Conroy
(486 NJA.2d 1209, 1985)

Claire Conroy was an 84-year-old, severely senile nursing home resident who was confined to her bed and fed through a nasogastric (NG) tube. Care takers were unable to communicate with her although she did show some response to the environment. Her nephew was her guardian and only living relative. He requested that the NG tube be withdrawn and his aunt allowed to die. Conroy had not, when competent, made her wishes regarding medical treatment known. The lower courts disagreed on whether it was permissible to withdraw the feeding tube, and the New Jersey Supreme Court heard the case. Conroy died prior to the decision.

The court established a complex set of guidelines under which feeding might be withheld. Their ruling applies, however, only to elderly, incompetent patients in nursing homes whose death can be anticipated within approximately one year. Feeding can be terminated if one of three conditions is met: if the person has specifically indicated while competent that such treatment is not desired, if the person has made general statements about not wanting treatment under such circumstances and the burdens of continuing treatment are greater than the benefits, or if the person has made no statement *and* the burdens of feedings "markedly and clearly" exceed the benefits.

In the last two conditions, the net burden of unavoidable pain must outweigh the benefits of staying alive. The *net burden* is the amount of unavoidable pain resulting from continuing feeding minus the unavoidable pain involved in dying from starvation. Pain alone is to be considered when determining the burdens of continued treatment and feeding. The court does not permit *substituted judgments* where there is no information about the patient's preferences. Only the *best interests* standard may be used. (Note that this is markedly different from the court's view in *Saikewicz*.) When the first, second, or third condition is believed to exist, the patient must be found incompetent and a guardian appointed. Then, the guardian, the physician, or the hospital must inform the state ombudsman of the desire to withhold food. The ombudsman must investigate the request as if it were a report of a "potential abuse" of an elderly person. Two disinterested physicians must be appointed to review the case and if they find the patient's medical prognosis to fall within the limits established by this decision and if the ombudsman finds that the

patient's situation meets one of the three conditions, then food can be withheld. A court does not need to be consulted. The court also found that there was insufficient evidence in the record to justify the withholding of food from Conroy.

This ruling, the first state supreme court ruling on withdrawing artificial feeding from incompetent but conscious patients, shows how concerned the courts are about potential abuses. The decision establishes strict protections for nursing home patients and applies only in a narrow range of circumstances. In fact, in the absence of the patient's having previously expressed specific preferences about not being fed under such conditions, it is possible that *no* patient will meet the guidelines, since pain can always be eliminated through adequate medication. Thus, if there is insufficient pain to *justify* withholding feeding, no withholding can occur unless the patient meets the first of the three conditions (specific preferences expressed when competent).

The importance of such forms as living wills and durable powers is demonstrated by this decision. The decision is binding only in New Jersey, of course, but other states' courts will probably take this decision into account when they are obliged to decide similar cases.

Foregoing Treatment: Competent Patients

Satz v. Perlmutter
(362 So.Rep.2d 160, 1978)

Abe Perlmutter was a 73-year-old patient with amyotrophic lateral sclerosis. Although respirator dependent, Perlmutter was fully competent. He requested that the respirator be disconnected but the hospital refused to permit this, fearing that it might be legally construed as homicide. The court weighed Perlmutter's right to refuse treatment against the state's interests in preserving life, protecting third parties, preventing suicide, and maintaining the integrity of medical practice.

The court discounted suicide on the grounds that it is an *unnatural* death, whereas disconnecting the respirator would lead to a *natural* death. The court found a further parallel between Perlmutter and terminally ill cancer patients who refuse therapy: in both, medical intervention only briefly postpones the inevitable. The state's interest in maintaining the integrity of the medical profession is not overridden by a decision to stop the respirator because current medical ethics recognizes that the dying patient may be more in need of comfort than of treatment. The court concluded that Perlmutter's right to refuse treatment should be honored. It further noted that the state legislature had failed to produce adequate legislation in this area and that fear of legal liability on the part of the hospital and the physicians could not be used to inflict further suffering on Perlmutter. To do so was to invade his right of privacy, his freedom of choice, and his right to self-determination.

Perlmutter is the kind of medical case that is often very troubling for both hospitals and courts, although in this particular case the court was very unambiguous about its conclusion. Although courts (and even health care providers) are nowadays often relatively comfortable with foregoing treatment for incompetent, comatose patients, it is psychologically much more difficult to stop treatment for a competent, conscious patient when the cessation will result in death. It appears that the patient's ability to function mentally has a greater claim on us and is thus valued more highly than biological life alone, as it is apparently exhibited by the comatose patient. Institutions, whether courts or hospitals, are very reluctant to acknowledge such views. *Perlmutter* strongly endorses privacy rights, even in the face of the discomfort created in those who must watch the patient die.

Bouvia v. County of Riverside, (Superior Ct., Riverside Co., CA, #159780, Dec. 16, 1983)[1]

Elizabeth Bouvia is a young woman who has had cerebral palsy from birth. She is able to control only her right hand and her facial muscles. Muscle contractures and arthritis have caused her to be in continual pain. She had graduated from college and married, but she was separated from her husband in 1983. In September of that year, she sought admission to Riverside General Hospital as a voluntary psychiatric patient. After her admission, she requested that she be permitted not to eat and that, while she died from starvation, the hospital provide her with nursing care and adequate pain medication. Her physicians refused and, when she refused to eat, the hospital announced its intention to force-feed her. Bouvia asked the court to prevent the forced feeding and to prohibit the hospital from discharging her as a patient.

The court determined that the plaintiff was competent and that her decision to end her life by refusing food was a rational one, born out of the extreme difficulties of her life, not from psychological depression resulting from her marital problems or her inability to find work. The court determined that the ultimate issue was "whether or not a severely handicapped, mentally competent person who is otherwise physically healthy and not mentally ill has the right to end her life with the assistance of society." The court concluded that she did not have such a right because, although a competent adult does have the right to terminate his or her life and to refuse life-saving medical treatment, in this case state and societal interests overcame that right. The state and societal interests cited by the judge included the state's interests in the preservation of life and the prevention of suicide. Assisting her to starve to death would be assisting her suicide, because her death was not otherwise imminent. The societal interests included those of the medical profession, whose ethics compelled them to preserve life, and the interests of other disabled individuals and patients within the hospital. The court then reasserted that Bouvia had the right to end her life, but she did not have the right to ask for societal—in this case medical—assistance when she was not terminally ill.

The court thus denied Bouvia's request to keep the hospital from discharging her or, if she remained as a patient, from feeding her by force or other means. The hospital was thus permitted, if Bouvia chose to remain there voluntarily, to force-feed her if she refused to eat.

Because this case was decided only at the superior court level, the ruling does not have significant *legal* force. The case does have enormous symbolic significance, however. This case arose during the same period that there was considerable publicity about the *Baby Doe* cases. In these cases, newborns with congenital anomalies were denied life-prolonging treatment, because their parents and physicians determined that their quality of life was too low. The *Bouvia* decision articulates the court's belief that handicapped persons' quality of life cannot be judged, either by themselves or by others, to be so low that health care professionals are obliged to participate actively in helping the person to die.

Bartling v. Superior Court (163 Cal.App.3d 186, 1984)

The *Bartling* decision reaffirms the central principle of medical decision making: competent patients have the moral and legal right to make their own treatment decisions, including both *consent* to and *refusal* of treatment.

Bartling was seriously ill when he entered the hospital but his death was not imminent. During a lung biopsy, his lung collapsed and he was placed on a ventilator. Both Bartling and his wife asked that the ventilator be removed. When the hospital and the treating physicians refused to comply with their request, Bartling appealed to the court.

The trial court stated that there was no precedent for discontinuing life support equipment when the patient was not comatose and terminally ill. On appeal, the California appellate court ruled that the trial court was wrong and that Bartling's right to refuse treatment was grounded in both the constitutional right of privacy and in California law. The court noted that California informed-consent cases clearly affirm the right of competent persons to control their own medical treatment and, further, that the California legislature, when passing the Natural Death Act, made a finding that adults have the right to control their own treatment.

The hospital argued that their interest in preserving life was central to their mission as a Christian prolife institution. The court responded that, if the patient's right to direct medical care is to be meaningful, it *must* outweigh the interests of the health care provider. (Note that this differs from the court's views of the hospital's obligations to perform abortions or sterilizations.)

In discussing the state's interest in preventing suicide, the court quoted the *Saikewicz* case. That decision said that a competent adult's refusal of medical treatment is not suicide because the patient may not have intended to die and, even if he did, death results from natural causes and not from something set in motion by the patient. If the patient's death is not a suicide, then the health care provider is not assisting a suicide. The *Bartling* decision specifically states that no civil or criminal liability follows when a health care provider complies with a competent patient's decision to refuse treatment. In addition, the court noted that prior judicial approval of such decisions was not legally required.

The *Bartling* decision reaffirms that the law gives precedence to individual autonomy. If conflicts between health care providers and competent patients cannot be resolved through dialogue, the patient's decision is determinative. (Note that this decision *appears* to conflict with the decision in the *Elizabeth Bouvia* case in which the hospital was permitted to feed her against her wishes. In that case, however, Bouvia did not have a terminal illness and feeding was not considered a form of treatment.)

Informed Consent

Canterbury v. Spence
(464 F.2d 772, 1972)

Canterbury was heard in the federal courts and the decision is that of a federal appellate court.

Canterbury consented to a laminectomy but his physician, Spence, did not inform him that permanent paralysis was a risk of the surgery. Canterbury did become paralyzed and sued Spence. The court found for Canterbury and the decision established, in the District of Columbia circuit, a patient's right to have adequate information to make a reasoned judgment about receiving medical treatment.

Prior to this case, the usual standard was customary or reasonable medical practice. The court found this standard inadequate because it gave greater weight to professional judgment than to individuals' right to make their own decisions (autonomy). The new standard established by this decision was that the patient should be told all he needed to know in order to make a reasoned judgment: "all risks potentially affecting the decision must be unmasked." The physician is expected to make a reasonable judgment about what would be of concern to the patient (including hazards of treatment, alternative treatments, and the results of no treatment). The court states that the physician should be found liable only when his standard of disclosure is "unreasonably inadequate."

The *Canterbury* standard for disclosure is "good law" in the federal courts of the Washington, DC, circuit. Informed consent cases, however, are much more likely to arise in state courts. Most states still continue to use customary professional practice as the standard for disclosure, although others have adopted the *Canterbury* standard.

Cobbs v. Grant (8 Cal.3d 229, 1972)

Cobbs v. Grant was decided by the California Supreme Court in 1972. The case involved a patient who consented to an operation for duodenal ulcer. The general risks of anesthesia were explained to him, but none of the possible complications or risks of the particular surgery were detailed. Cobbs underwent three subsequent hospital admissions: for a splenectomy, as the result of a severed artery at the hilum of the spleen; for a gastrectomy following development of a gastric ulcer; and for treatment of internal bleeding as a result of a prematurely absorbed suture. All were known risks of the surgery.

When the California Supreme Court decided the case, they gave specific instructions as to how the issue of informed consent should be handled. Failure to gain consent for medical treatment (in nonemergency situations) constitutes battery. Failure to provide adequate disclosure of information necessary to ensure informed consent, on the other hand, is negligence. Like the *Canterbury* court, the *Cobbs* court held that the patient's right to exercise control over his own body and make reasonable decisions was primary. In order to exercise control, the patient must have "all information relevant to a meaningful decisional process." In the context of complex procedures like the surgery in question, the court specifically states that inherent risks of death or serious bodily injuries must be revealed.

Sterilization

Many states do not permit sterilization of incompetent patients. In other states, legislatures have established by statute specific procedures to authorize sterilization of incompetents. Because of the wide-scale abuse of sterilization that occurred in the first half of this century in the wake of the eugenics movement, these consent procedures are drawn very narrowly and are usually quite restrictive. In the absence of specific legislation, courts will seldom authorize sterilization of an incompetent patient.

Ruby v. Massey (452 F.Supp. 361, 1978)

This case was brought by three sets of parents of three severely retarded and physically handicapped teenagers. The parents wished to consent to hysterectomies for their respective daughters but Connecticut, like many states, does not permit parental consent for sterilization of incompetents. Connecticut had, however, established a special procedure to authorize sterilization for incompetent patients in two state institutions. The minors in this case were not residents of either institution. In this case, the federal district court found that providing consent procedures to sterilization for some incompetent patients but denying them to others was discriminatory and thus a denial of due process.

Ruby is not a uniquely important case in itself, but it is representative of the many legal problems involved in sterilization in the light of the constitutionally protected right to procreation. In abortion cases, the Supreme Court has ruled that hospitals need not provide abortion services if they choose not to. Hospital refusal to perform sterilizations would very likely be handled in the same way so long as all parties were treated similarly (that is, as long as the policy did not discriminate in some way).

Wrongful Life

For many years, wrongful life suits were rejected in every jurisdiction, usually because, as the courts claimed, it was impossible to say that no life was better than being born with disabilities. In recent years, however, courts are beginning to accept these cases, although many state courts have continued to reject all suits involving wrongful life. (Note the distinction between *wrongful birth* and *wrongful life*. Wrongful birth involves the parents' claim that a birth should not have happened; wrongful life involves the *child's* claim that it should not have been born.)

Curlender v. Bioscience Laboratories (106 Cal.App.3d 811, 1980)

The Curlenders sought testing to determine if they were Tay-Sachs disease carriers and were informed that they were not carriers. This information was incorrect, and their child was born with Tay-Sachs disease. In this suit, the infant was claiming damages on the grounds that she had been injured by being born. This action is frequently called wrongful life. (It should be noted that this is different from wrongful birth, a claim that is made by the parents. A wrongful birth claim was also made in *Curlender*.) The case came to the appellate court on the question of whether it presented a legitimate *cause of action*. That is, if the facts were as the plaintiffs said they were, did that constitute a *legal* wrong?

A number of similar complaints had been filed in courts across the United States since the mid-1970s. These included cases in which Down's syndrome infants were born to parents-at-risk, who had not been informed of the risk or of the availability of amniocentesis; cases of infants with hereditary diseases in which parents had either not been told of the risk or had been told there was no risk; and cases in which testing for the genetic defect had been performed but the tests had provided incorrect answers. In these cases, the parents usually were awarded damages (wrongful birth) for their own costs or for costs of the handicapped child's care. In none of these cases was the child awarded damages. The claim was made that the infant had and would suffer pain and emotional distress as a result of being born so severely handicapped. The courts, however, agreed that except for the defendant's negligence, the child would not have been born at all. Thus, to award damages to the child was the equivalent of saying the child should never have been born and that no life was better than an impaired life. Such a statement, according to these courts, violated public policy.

When the California appellate court heard the *Curlender* case, the decision was made against this background. None of these other cases was heard in California so the court was not bound by precedent.

The California appellate court upheld the infant's wrongful life claim in *Curlender* and, thus, became the first court in the United States to say that wrongful life was a legally recognizable cause of action. The decision argued that it was wrong to combine the child's birth and the child's handicap, as was done by previous courts. That is, other courts had argued that the only alternative action to the handicap was not being born. Although true, the California court said, the infant *had* been born and had suffered an injury that should be redressed in this life. On the other hand, the child should not receive damages measured against a normal life, but only in terms of its actual life. Thus, a seriously shortened life could not be taken into consideration. The California Supreme Court declined to hear the case.

The issues of wrongful life are philosophically and legally difficult. The many courts that denied these claims were concerned about a general devaluing of the life of the handicapped (that is, that they were better off dead), as well as a fear that it would open the way to handicapped children suing their parents for giving birth to them. In the wake of the California decision, the state legislature passed a law prohibiting wrongful life suits by children against parents.

Note

1. In 1986, the California appellate court held that Ms. Bouvia was entitled to refuse the nasogastric tube feedings recommended by her physician. Many disagree about whether this decision, which affirmed a competent patient's right to refuse treatment, means that a patient can commit suicide by refusing treatment. The California Supreme Court declined to review the case (*Bouvia v. Superior Court of Los Angeles*), No. B 019134, April 16, 1986).

Appendixes

Appendixes A, B, and C were reprinted with permission from the following sources:

Appendix A
American Hospital Association, Chicago
American Medical Association, Chicago

Appendix B
Abbott Northwestern Hospital, Minneapolis
Metropolitan Medical Center, Minneapolis
Lovelace Medical Center, Albuquerque, NM
St. Joseph Hospital, Orange, CA
Rose Medical Center, Denver
St. Paul-Ramsey Medical Center, St. Paul

Appendix C
Presbyterian Healthcare Services, Albuquerque, NM
St. Joseph Hospital, Orange, CA
St. Paul-Ramsey Medical Center, St. Paul

Appendix A

Guidelines for Ethics Committees

American Hospital Association
Guidelines: Hospital Committees on Biomedical Ethics

Introduction

The growth of medical knowledge and the rapid expansion of medical capabilities and technology have generated unprecedented opportunities and challenges in the delivery of health care. At the same time, this growth and expansion have created increasingly complex ethical choices for physicians, health care professionals, patients, and the families of patients. Recent efforts to clarify biomedical ethical issues on the institutional level have focused on the use of hospital biomedical ethics committees. Such committees, sometimes called "ethics committees," "human values committees," "medical-moral committees," or "bioethics committees," hold promise for identifying the ethical implications of these problems and their possibile resolutions, if they are established with a clearly defined purpose and an understanding of their capabilities and limitations.

Institutional ethics committees are one of several approaches to address medical ethical matters. If an institution chooses this approach, the following guidelines may assist in determining the organization, composition, and function of these committees. Because such committees are relatively new and largely untested, the guidelines are not intended to be prescriptive or directive.

Functions

Although institutional ethics committees may have one or more functions, they seem particularly suited to:(1) directing educational programs on biomedical ethical issues, (2) providing forums for discussion among hospital and medical professionals and others about biomedical ethical issues, (3) serving in an advisory capacity and/or as a resource to persons involved in biomedical decision making, and (4) evaluating institutional experiences related to reviewing decisions having biomedical ethical implications. Ethics committees should not serve as professional ethics review boards, as substitutes for legal or judicial review, or as "decision makers" in biomedical ethical dilemmas. An ethics committee should not replace the traditional loci of decision making on these issues.

Educational programs on biomedical ethics issues serve to heighten awareness and provide guidance on identification of cases where ethical problems may arise. Such programs may be offered to medical staff, the hospital staff, and the community. Forums for the discussion of these issues serve similar purposes by providing an opportunity for physicians, nurses, administrators, trustees, clergy, ethicists, and others to consider and discuss a number of diverse perspectives.

The use of ethics committees in an advisory role to assist physicians, other health care professionals, and patients and their families to make decisions when confronted with

Reprinted, with permission, from American Hospital Association. AHA Copyright 1984.

This guideline document is intended to provide general advice to the membership of the American Hospital Association, as approved by the General Council. The American Hospital Association's General Council created a Special Committee on Biomedical Ethics in 1982. This multidisciplinary committee prepared these guidelines as part of its charge to assist hospitals in developing institutional processes to deal with the educational and decision-making challenges presented by biomedical ethical issues. These guidelines were approved by the AHA General Council on January 27, 1984.

dilemmas is probably their most complex function. Ethics committees often may make recommendations at the request of an attending physician, another hospital professional closely connected with the case, the hospital administration, and the patient or the patient's family. Access to the committee should be open to all those involved in patient care decisions. Hospitals should design and implement systems to bring to the committee's attention certain kinds of issues and to address similar issues in a reasonably consistent manner.

Composition

The members of an ethics committee should be selected in keeping with its objectives and represent a range of perspectives and expertise. It may be multidisciplinary and may include physicians, nurses, administrators, social workers, clergy, trustees, attorneys, ethicists, and patient advocates (representatives). Hospital legal counsel should be available at the request of the committee, and legal review of its recommendations may be necessary.

To be most useful and effective, an ethics committee should be a standing committee, and its members should be approved by the appropriate authority within the institution. This structure provides continuity and enhances the credibility of the committee. It also provides an opportunity for the committee to develop an understanding of the permissible range for discretion and latitude within which biomedical ethical decisions may be made. The committee should meet regularly and whenever necessary to provide advice and recommendations. As a general rule, no one who is personally involved in the case in question should serve on the committee while the case is being considered.

Deliberations

Issues that may be brought to an ethics committee acting in an advisory capacity should relate to patient care.

If a recommendation is made by the committee, it should be provided as appropriate to the physicians, nurses, and other health care professionals involved in treatment, and should be offered to the patient and the patient's family or other surrogate.

The confidentiality of patient information and the patient's privacy should be respected. The circumstances under which documentation of the committee's recommendations should appear in the patient's medical records should be determined by each institution with the advice of legal counsel.

The manner in which the committee considers an issue or a particular case should depend on the individual circumstances. The committee may review and discuss materials submitted to it, or it may meet with the health care team involved and others as needed, including persons acting on the patient's behalf.

Conclusion

Each institution should take the steps necessary to implement suitable mechanisms that will reasonably provide for sound decision-making practices and for responsible and timely assessment of medical and ethical issues.

American Medical Association Guidelines for Ethics Committees in Health Care Institutions

These guidelines have been developed to aid in the establishment and functioning of ethics committees in hospitals and other health care institutions that may choose to form such committees, recognizing that the functions may vary depending on the type of institution.

Ethics committees in health care institutions should be voluntary, educational, and advisory in purpose so as not to interfere with the primary responsibility and relationship between physicians and their patients. Generally, the function of the ethics committee is to consider and assist in resolving unusual, complicated ethical problems involving issues that affect the care and treatment of patients within the health care institution and concern those persons who are responsible for their care and treatment. Typical are issues involving quality of life, terminal illness, and utilization of scarce, limited health resources.

The size of the ethics committee should be consistent with the needs of the institution but not so large in number as to be unwieldy. Members of the committee should be selected on the basis of their concern for the welfare of the sick and infirm, their interest in ethical matters, and their reputation in the community and among their peers for integrity and mature judgment. Preferably, a majority of the committee should consist of physicians, nurses, and other health care providers.

Persons considered for the ethics committee should be temperamentally suited to making recommendations affecting the welfare of patients and professional considerations relating to their care and treatment. Experience as a member of hospital or medical society committees concerned with ethical conduct or quality assurance should be given weight in selecting members of the committee. It is important that persons selected as committee members should not have other responsibilities that are likely to prove incompatible with their duties as members of the ethics committee.

The functions of the ethics committee should be confined exclusively to ethical matters. In hospitals, the medical staff bylaws should delineate the functions of the ethics committee, general qualifications for membership, manner of selection, and parameters of the committee's activities. The *Principles of Medical Ethics* and *Current Opinions of the Judicial Council of the American Medical Association* are recommended for the guidance of ethics committees in the making of their own recommendations.

Although the recommendations that the ethics committee may make may involve the application of moral standards that exceed those imposed by law, such recommendations should not contravene or violate applicable laws of the jurisdiction or call upon others to do so. In denominational health care institutions or those operated by religious orders, the recommendations of the ethics committee may be anticipated to be consistent with published religious tenets and principles. Where particular religious beliefs are to be taken into consideration in the committee's recommendation, this fact should be publicized to those persons concerned with the committee's recommendations.

Reprinted, with permission, from the Judicial Council, American Medical Association.

Presented to the House of Delegates in Judicial Council Report E, which was adopted by the House at the December 1984 Interim Meeting.

The matters to be considered by the ethics committee should consist of ethical subjects that a majority of its members may choose to discuss on its own initiative, matters referred to it by the executive committee of the organized medical staff or by the governing board of the institution, or appropriate requests from patients, families of patients, or physicians. The ethics committee may also choose to consider requests from other health professionals who are employed by the institution and who pursue the matter through designated appropriate administrative channels.

Generally, recommendations of the ethics committee should be in writing and channeled through the executive committee of the organized medical staff for consideration of those persons who may have a direct interest in the committee's recommendations. In the absence of an organized medical staff, the committee's recommendations should be channeled through the administrator of the institution or the latter's designee. The procedures followed by the ethics committee should comply with institutional policies for preserving the confidentiality of information regarding patients.

The recommendations of the ethics committee should be offered precisely as recommendations imposing no obligation for acceptance on the part of the institution, its governing board, medical staff, attending physician, or other persons. On the other hand, it is expected that the ethics committee will give patient consideration and sympathetic understanding to matters that it is called upon to study, and that the institution will provide the committee with necessary staff assistance. Typically, it should be expected that the efforts of a dedicated committee will receive serious consideration by those whose responsibility it is to function as decision makers.

Those who are selected as members of the ethics committee should be prepared to meet on short notice and to render their recommendations in a timely and prompt fashion in accordance with the demands of the situation and the issues involved.

Additional Reading

Infant Bioethics Task Force and Consultants. Guidelines for Infant Bioethics Committees. *Pediatrics.* 1984. 74(2):306-310.

Federal Register. Services and Treatment for Disabled Infants: Model Guidelines for Health Care Providers to Establish Infant Care Review Committees. April 15, 1985. 50(72): 14893-14900.

Appendix **B**

Committee Function and Goal Statements

Abbott Northwestern Hospital
Minneapolis, MN
Ethical and Moral Values in Health Care

Mission Statement

Abbott-Northwestern Hospital is committed to the care of people from birth through death, in a manner that insures patient and family dignity, privacy, and respect. We affirm the right of the patient to participate in the planning and decision-making process affecting his or her treatment. These rights are facilitated by the hospital providing a consultation team and individual/family counseling services.

Abbott-Northwestern Hospital is committed to the support and education of employees and physicians in biomedical ethics and the process of biomedical ethical decision-making. Commitment is demonstrated through the provision of a consultation team, educational activities, and employee counseling services, so that the employee and physician may be an active participant in the ethic process in either a professional or personal situation.

Consultation

A consultation team is available to deal with biomedical ethical issues on behalf of patient, family, and health team members. The consultation team provides a forum through which:

- the rights of patients, family, and health team members are clarified
- issues are discussed, clarified, and mediated
- biomedical ethical issues are considered in the context of costs and reimbursement constraints
- support is offered to involved decision-makers

The consultation team will serve patients/families and staff throughout LifeSpan Inc. Patients, family, and health team members request the services of the team through the attending physician. The attending physician(s) and nurse(s) should participate in the consultation. The physician is responsible for recording discussion and/or consensus in the medical record, when indicated. Consultation team members are selected on the basis of their clinical specialty and experience with ethical issues from among physicians, nurses, social workers, patient representatives, chaplains, and consumers. Additional members serve according to individual situations. Members are expected to maintain current knowledge regarding the field of ethics.

Education

An education committee is appointed by the steering committee on ethical and moral values in health care. The education committee will assess educational needs specific to biomedical ethics of hospital staff and physicians, and plan educational activities to meet assessed needs. The education committee will plan and lead the monthly ethics conference. An evaluation of educational activities will be completed annually.

Counseling

Counseling services for patients/families, employees, and physicians are available through multiple hospital departments and services. Services are provided on an individual basis or through group processes. Hospital staff and physicians can assist patients/families in selecting the service most appropriate to their needs.

Metropolitan Medical Center
A HealthOne Company
Minneapolis, MN

Advisory Committee on Ethical Decision Making

General Statement

Metropolitan Medical Center's Medical Staff has a Committee on Ethical Decision Making. Resources of this committee are available to all patients and their families through their medical doctors.

How to Request Help

You should speak directly with your doctor about decisions being made about your health care. If you are uncertain about the issues, your nurse, patient representative, social worker, or chaplain will be happy to assist you in discussing any concerns.

Purpose of the Advisory Committee on Ethical Decision Making

A. *TO* promote and facilitate communication and sharing of information so mutual understanding between health care providers and receivers is achieved

B. *TO* address any ethical dilemma(s)

C. *TO* support patients and their loved ones who face issues regarding treatment and prognosis. As there is need for all health care providers to have a place to discuss ideas and emotions about patient care:

   1. The consultation service will be available for the purpose of discussion and support.
   2. In these cases, it shall be made clear that this is not a consultation to the patient or medical staff.

D. *TO* assist staff in clarifying treatment goals and care plans

E. *TO* include clinical judgment in considering problems, supporting patients and staff, and evaluating the consultation process

Lovelace Medical Center
Albuquerque, NM
Bylaw

Article XI — Medical Ethics Advisory Committee

A. *Composition:* Membership shall consist of representatives of the medical and nursing staff, Center administration, hospital chaplain, legal profession, and the lay community. A representative of a disability group or a developmental disability expert shall serve as a full member when the committee is serving as an Infant Care Review Committee (ICRC). The chairperson shall be empowered to appoint temporary ad hoc members whose expertise may be necessary for a particular issue. Membership shall not normally exceed ten members. Because of the sensitive nature of deliberations, the committee may establish rules to preserve confidentiality.

B. *Duties:* The Medical Ethics Advisory Committee shall serve as an advisory body when medical ethics issues are encountered by the professional or administrative staff. It shall also serve the function of an ICRC where mandated by law.

Additional functions include the following:

1. Education of professional staff in current medical-ethical concepts
2. Development of ethical guidelines that enhance the quality of patient care
3. Advice to other staff committees
4. Advice upon request of providers faced with difficult ethical issues in individual patient care. Such advice shall not replace the ultimate responsibility of the attending physician in such matters

Saint Joseph Hospital
Orange, California

Perinatal Bioethics Committee Bylaws

I. Purpose

The purpose of the Perinatal Bioethics Committee shall be to serve as an advisory body to the hospital's medical and administrative staff on matters relating to moral and ethical decisions presented while rendering care and treatment in the perinatal field.

II. Objectives

A. *Education*

1. To provide a forum for the discussion of ethical questions and concerns that arise in the hospital regarding perinatal matters and are not addressed systematically by other committees
2. To encourage and assist in the development of bioethical education programs consisting of conferences and medical library resource materials
3. To monitor state and federal legislation for ethical implications and make appropriate responses

B. *Policy and Guideline Development*

To serve as an advisory body for administrative and professional staffs on the formulation of policies and/or guidelines concerned with ethical issues in perinatal care

C. *Case Review*

1. The committee may review the care of a patient upon the request of any member of the hospital staff or member of the patient's immediate family when an ethical issue is presented concerning the patient's care.
2. The committee may review any case of a hospitalized infant or mother when ethical questions about the patient's care have been raised by a public agency.
3. The committee should review all cases in which there is serious disagreement among the staff responsible for the care of a patient or patients or between the attending physician and the parents of an infant patient.
4. The committee shall make a retrospective review of all cases in which the attending physician and the parents have elected to forego, by withholding or withdrawing, life-sustaining treatment for an infant.

The above is an excerpt from the bylaws.

Rose Medical Center
Denver, CO

Ethics and Human Values Committee Bylaws

Article I. *Name: Ethics and Human Values Committee*

Article II. *Purpose, Goals, and Functions*

Section 1. Purpose: To foster awareness of ethical issues in the hospital environment.

Section 2. Goals:

A. To aid in formulating hospital policy concerning medical-ethical issues
B. To provide a nonjudgmental atmosphere in which to explore ethical dilemmas, both prospectively and retrospectively, by clarification of values and development of rational decision-making processes for a pluralistic society
C. To serve as a forum and source of ideas for resolution of ethical conflict in actual hospital cases

Section 3. Functions:

The Committee:

A. Can be called upon for consultation regarding ethical issues by medical and paramedical hospital staff, administrators, patients, families, or the public and duly constituted civic authorities
B. May initiate examination of policy or practice in order to further its stated purpose
C. May utilize hospital resources for programs to promote its purpose, but participation by staff or patients is wholly voluntary
D. Will have no decision-making function nor any enforcement power for its recommendations aside from existing hospital processes, as stated in hospital bylaws
E. Will provide resources for the general education of hospital medical and paramedical staff

---

The above is an excerpt from the bylaws.

Bioethics Consultation Subcommittee
St. Paul-Ramsey Medical Center, St. Paul, MN
Consultation Subcommittee Guidelines

Goals

1. Respond to requests for biomedical ethics consultations for patients of SPRMC
2. Continually inform and educate subcommittee members of current biomedical ethical issues and problems
3. Maintain a forum for discussion and review of consultations and bioethical concerns

Membership

Persons interested in devoting time and effort in achieving goals of the subcommittee. Included but not limited to this group will be the following: chaplain, ethicist, nurse, physician, social worker, patient representative. Ex officio members will include an administrative representative and legal counsel. Members are expected to attend the monthly meetings of the Hospital Bioethics Committee and also the scheduled consultation subcommittee meetings. Members of this subcommittee will also respond to consultation requests. Members are expected to make a 2 to 3 year commitment to this subcommittee.

At the end of the year the subcommittee will review its composition and discuss officers.

Meetings

The consultation subcommittee will meet at least monthly and by request.

Consultation Procedure

1. Initiation—Request for consultation may come at any time from any individual who is concerned about an existing or potential ethical dilemma for a patient. The initiator should contact the chairperson or any other member of the subcommittee.
2. Triage—If the chairperson was not initially contacted, the subcommittee member involved will notify the chairperson. One or more members will then assess the circumstances by discussion with the initiator, others involved, and review of the patient chart. If ethical issues are identified, a formal consultation will follow.
3. The attending physician will be notified of the consultation either by the consult team or the initiator.
4. Formal consultation—The consultation may be provided by:

   A. The triage team or,
   B. The triage team plus subcommittee members, as needed.

   1. Whenever possible, the consultation team shall include but not be limited to representatives of pastoral care, nursing, physician, social work, administration, and ethicist.
   2. In a given case, the primary care givers' participation in the discussion is essential. However, a primary care giver will not sit as a member of the consultation team.

Consultation Process

1. Process for consultation will follow the general outline below:

    A. Collection of data base
    B. Case presentation
    C. Identification of medical problems
    D. Identification of psychosocial problems
    E. Identification of ethical problems
    F. Identification of legal issues
    G. Discussion of ethical issues
    H. Suggestions for approaches to the problems
    I. Discussion with initiator, patient, if possible, and other involved individuals not present at consultation meeting
    J. Documentation of issues discussed and suggested approaches will be placed in the patient's chart. Written summaries of the consultation will be filed

2. The subcommittee does not make patient care decisions.
3. Each consultation will be reviewed and discussed at the monthly subcommittee meeting.

Miscellaneous

These guidelines will be reviewed annually.

Appendix **C**

Consultation Forms

Presbyterian Healthcare Services
Albuquerque, New Mexico

Record of Consultation by Quality of Life Committee
(To be attached to copy of Admission Record)

Consultation requested by: _____

Date: _____   Time: _____

Reason for consultation:

_____

_____

Attending physician notified by: _____

Date: _____   Time: _____

Comments: _____

Date of consultation: _____   Time: _____

Consultants:

_____   _____

_____   _____

_____   _____

Patient and/or family members present:

_____   _____

_____   _____

Brief summary: _____

_____

_____

Follow-up: _____   Time: _____

_____

_____

Saint Joseph Hospital
Orange, CA

Bioethics Committee
Record of Patient Review Session

Patient medical record number: _____

>At the start of a patient review session, a member of the Bioethics Committee will open the meeting by reminding those present that

- The ensuing discussion will be held in confidence
- Decisions regarding medical care of the patient remain with the physician/patient/family
- It is accepted that agreement/concensus may not occur
- A report of this review session will be sent to the physicians involved; Bioethics Committee members will view the report for educational purposes only

Date of review: _____

Those present:

_____   _____

_____   _____

_____   _____

_____   _____

_____   _____

Dilemma and/or situation (do not identify patient or anyone else by name):

_____

_____

_____

_____

_____

Questions addressed:

_____

_____

_____

_____

_____

_____

Questions addressed: (continued)

_____

_____

_____

_____

_____

_____

_____

Recommendations:

A. Suggestions regarding care surrounding patient

_____

_____

_____

_____

_____

_____

_____

B. Hospital policy/procedure changes

_____

_____

_____

_____

_____

_____

_____

_____

_____

_____

_____

_____

When complete, forward to the secretary of the Bioethics Committee.

St. Paul-Ramsey Medical Center
St. Paul, MN

Bioethics Consultation Subcommittee
Evaluation Form

The members of the Bioethics Consultation Subcommittee wish to know if their responses to your consult have been timely, helpful, and effective. In order to constantly improve the service offered, we need feedback. Your response to the following questionnaire is essential. Thank you.

Please check the number that most clearly reflects your opinion.

1	2	3	4	5
Strongly agree		Neutral		Strongly disagree

1. The team of professionals who responded to your request

    A. Were open to your concerns   A. | 1 | 2 | 3 | 4 | 5 |

    B. Asked useful questions   B. | 1 | 2 | 3 | 4 | 5 |

    C. Clarified issues   C. | 1 | 2 | 3 | 4 | 5 |

    D. Seemed knowledgeable   D. | 1 | 2 | 3 | 4 | 5 |

    E. Assisted in the process   E. | 1 | 2 | 3 | 4 | 5 |

    Comments: _____

    _____

    _____

2. The consultation note:

    A. Addressed issues raised   A. | 1 | 2 | 3 | 4 | 5 |

    B. Offered helpful approaches   B. | 1 | 2 | 3 | 4 | 5 |

    C. Was clear   C. | 1 | 2 | 3 | 4 | 5 |

    D. Contributed nothing new   D. | 1 | 2 | 3 | 4 | 5 |

    Comments: _____

    _____

    _____

3. As a result of the consult:

    A. Ethical issues were clarified   A. | 1 | 2 | 3 | 4 | 5 |

    B. Your decision making was facilitated   B. | 1 | 2 | 3 | 4 | 5 |

    C. You became aware of additional perspectives   C. | 1 | 2 | 3 | 4 | 5 |

    D. You had increased confidence in your patient
        care decisions   D. | 1 | 2 | 3 | 4 | 5 |

    Comments _____

    _____

    _____

4. The consultation provided an opportunity for
health professionals to express concerns, raise questions, give input, and receive explanations. | 1 | 2 | 3 | 4 | 5 |

    Comments:_____

    _____

5. The response was prompt. | 1 | 2 | 3 | 4 | 5 |

    Comments:_____

6. The consult team was easily acessible.   [ ] Yes   [ ] No

    Comments:_____

7. As a result of your experience, are you more likely
or less likely to seek the assistance of the Bioethics
Consultation Subcommittee again?   [ ] more likely

                                           [ ] less likely

    Comments:_____

8. Have you any additional remarks for the
committee?   [ ] Yes   [ ] No

    Explain: _____

    _____   Signed _____
                                                             optional

Please return to: Chairman
                      Bioethics Consultation Subcommittee
                      Medicine Department

Appendix **D**

Group Leadership

To help ethics committees work as a group, we have assembled some practical suggestions from our own experience and from a program entitled "Group Action."[1]

Managing Meetings

A group leader needs to consider three major areas of organization: getting the meeting started, keeping it moving, and generating action.

Getting the Meeting Started

Well before the meeting begins, the group leader needs to define the purpose of the meeting, create an agenda, and let the participants know why the meeting is to be held.

- *Defining the purpose and desired outcomes.* This is a crucial first step. Many meetings wander, struggle, and eventually fail because it was not clear to begin with where they were going. The group leader should determine why the meeting is being called (purpose) and what it is intended to accomplish or achieve (objectives). This step is more difficult to determine with a routinely scheduled meeting, but it can be combined with creating the agenda.
- *Creating the meeting agenda.* The agenda is an important tool for a well-managed meeting. If developed conscientiously, it serves as a map to keep the meeting on track and on time. Consider the following questions when developing the agenda:
  —What are the topics to be discussed?
  —What should be accomplished with each topic?
  —Who is responsible for each topic?
  —What are participants expected to do? Contribute information? Make recommendations? Give commitment? Give feedback? Approve?
  —How much time will you allow for each topic? Some meetings may require time limits on each agenda item, whereas other meetings may not require such structure. The group leader needs to review the purpose and objectives of the meeting to determine whether time limits are necessary.
  —Which topic has priority? Generally, the most important items should be discussed first, particularly if time is limited.
- *Communicating the purpose and desired outcome to all participants.* Although this sounds obvious, it is often overlooked. The easiest way of communicating the purpose and plan of the meeting is to mail the agenda, along with all the documents

that need to be read ahead of time. This also serves as a reminder to the participants of the meeting time and place. If the meeting is scheduled at a regular time, this should be mailed out about a week ahead of time. If meeting times are irregular, it may need to be mailed earlier.

Keeping the Meeting Moving

Many groups work together to perform a task (athletes on a team or actors in a play). In any such group activity, the activity proceeds best when someone — the coach, the director — is standing back, watching the overall workings of the group. A group leader needs to fulfill the same function, but sometimes the leader becomes so involved in the discussion that he or she loses track of the process. If no one is watching the big picture, that is, managing the meeting, the meeting is unlikely to achieve its objectives. A good leader needs to learn how to attend to both content and process. The following steps will help in that goal.

- *Reviewing the meeting agenda.* This important first step focuses the participants' attention on the task at hand. It is also a good time to ask for any changes or additions to the agenda. If the meeting has been called for a specific purpose and desired outcome (as opposed to a routinely scheduled meeting), take time to restate the purpose and objectives of the meeting. If time limits are listed on the agenda, the committee should determine how they will handle a discussion that requires more than the allotted time. (The committee might agree, in advance, to table the discussion for a later meeting, or to continue the discussion and table other agenda items.)
- *Defining or reviewing the ground rules for the meeting.* This will depend on the nature of the meeting and of the group. Ground rules are used to state expectations regarding behavior. They give members guidance on the kind of participation desired. Ground rules also allow members to confront unacceptable behavior. For a newly established group, the leader will have to create the ground rules. For a well-established group, little time may be required for reviewing the rules at each meeting. Typically, ground rules pertain to the kind of participation expected, the kind of behavior expected (that is, no put-downs, sharing discussion time equally, listening without interruptions), nonnegotiable matters (time limits, if applicable), confidentiality, money constraints (if applicable), and role assignments (recorder, timekeeper).

- *Focusing the discussion on the purpose and the desired outcome.* Much time is wasted in meetings because irrelevant information is dumped into them. Everyone has been in a meeting where the group has wandered from one topic to another. Fundamental to the meeting's effectiveness is keeping the purpose and objectives of the meeting or a given agenda item in front of the group. In order to prevent this wandering, determine if the discussion is off target. Is it drifting off into left field? Is related but irrelevant information being introduced? Is the storytelling appropriate? Is the debate focusing on trivia? Is the discussion moving from point to point without resolution? If so, then it is time to refocus the discussion. This takes great skill on the part of the group leader. It is necessary to evaluate the discussion carefully—by refocusing too quickly, participation is stifled; by waiting too long, control (as well as time) is lost. When redirecting the discussion, the group leader should ask questions and make statements that will lead the discussion back to the objectives of the specific agenda topic or to the general purpose of the meeting.
- *Setting the pace.* Even when the discussion is focused on the objective, it must move at an appropriate pace. Conclusions reached too quickly and discussions that never end are two sides of the same problem. The meeting may be too slow if the group is groping for ideas or recommendations, if information and ideas are being rehashed, if energy levels are dropping, or if the participants seem bored. The meeting may be moving too fast if conclusions are reached rapidly with little discussion, if not everyone has sufficient opportunity to give opinions or to ask questions, or if not enough data have been generated.
- *Articulating conclusions.* Productive meetings occur when conclusions are reached throughout the meeting. If conclusions are articulated only at the very end, ideas are often forgotten or lost and participants may then disagree about what was decided. Thus, it is more effective to reach conclusions at the following times:
  - After each major topic or item is considered
  - After all relevant information has been presented
  - After all sides of an issue have been expressed
  - When the group decides it is ready to make a decision

Generating Action at a Meeting

An accurate description of many meetings might be, "When all is said and done, a lot more is said than done." Frequently a group leader is so relieved that a decision appears to have been reached that no implementation plans are made. Everyone concurs so the group moves on to the next topic. In other situations, the leader makes quick plans without adequate thought to the steps needed or the appropriate persons to carry out the task. In order to avoid this, it is helpful to create an action plan after each conclusion is reached. Members then leave the meeting feeling that they have accomplished something and that there will be follow-through. In order to create an action plan, it is helpful to:

- Specify what action needs to be taken
- Make specific assignments with completion dates
- Agree on how to monitor progress and/or evaluate outcomes

Leadership Skills

In addition to being able to organize and manage the process of a meeting, a group leader also needs to have personal leadership skills. These focus on handling behavior that is key to group interaction. The leader needs to give special attention to encouraging participation, handling disruptive behavior, and managing diversity.

Encouraging Participation

The leader's behavior usually determines group participation. Effective leaders see their role as coach or conductor of the group, and to fill that role, they need to understand something about the individual feelings and expectations of the participants. Some people are very cautious and hesitate to contribute anything until they are absolutely certain they understand everything that is going on. Some participants simply do not have the kind of assertive behavior that allows them to contribute. Others feel that contributing their ideas may invite criticism. Effective group leaders need to look actively for ways to draw out such participants.

- *Specifying the type of participation that is desired.* By clearly stating the type of participation desired for any agenda topic, the group leader prevents any misconceptions and keeps the meeting focused. Some of the types of participation that may be appropriate are clarifications, questions, discussion, generation of ideas or alternatives, analysis, decisions, and feedback.
- *Creating a participatory climate.* People respond to the climate around them. Open, inviting climates

encourage participation. To create a participatory climate, the group leader may want to hold back in order to provide time for others to talk, to save his or her opinion until the end, to maintain a receptive and informal atmosphere, to ask open-ended questions, and to discourage frequent participant-to-leader dialogue. Attention should be focused on the topic, not on the leader. If participants direct comments primarily to the leader, the leader should turn them back to the group.

- *Drawing out contributions from specific individuals.* To obtain full participation, a leader often has to make specific overtures to individuals to encourage their participation. To miss a person's contribution can be unproductive for everyone. Contributions can often be drawn out by directing questions to individuals rather than to the total group and by seeking out the uninvolved.
- *Protecting persons with minority views.* Asserting the value of everyone's viewpoint is important because a variety of approaches and perspectives encourages creative thinking. It also lets people know the group is open to ideas.
- *Acknowledging and reinforcing constructive participation.* People repeat what has been reinforced. Without acknowledgment, participation is likely to decrease. Participation can be encouraged by giving both verbal and nonverbal reinforcement (good idea, thanks for pointing that out, that's an important consideration, nodding, keeping eye contact, and so on), by encouraging the expression of partial ideas, and by collectively acknowledging the group's achievements.

Handling Disruptive Behavior

Disruptive behavior is generally unintentional. Nevertheless, it can seriously inhibit the group's progress. It diverts discussion from the real agenda. If the meeting is to be successful the leader must stop disruptive behavior before it interferes with the group process. How it is stopped is crucial. An effective leader learns how to stop disruptive behavior without embarrassing those involved, without creating an uncomfortable situation, and without inhibiting participation. Examples of disruptive behavior might include:

- Bringing unrelated subjects into the discussion
- Discouraging group action by saying, "This will never work," or, "There is no solution to this problem"
- Dominating the discussion and preventing others from contributing

- Interrupting others
- Disagreeing with everyone

The group's leader should take steps to minimize disruptive behavior. He or she should not assume that the behavior is deliberate. Often people do not recognize that their actions are blocking group progress. Leaders might try the following guidelines to minimize disruptions:

- Remain calm. Personal anger or irritation should not be expressed, though firmness and promptness is necessary. The least disruptive action that will correct the problem should be used. If subtle suggestions do not work, then stronger measures are needed.
- Summarize or clarify. Sometimes the meeting and the discussion can be refocused by clarifying what was going on before the disruptive behavior began.
- Refer to the ground rules.
- Use nonverbal behavior.
- Make a direct statement to the person or persons involved. There are instances where nothing works except direct verbal confrontation. Remember to focus on the *behavior* that is disruptive, not on the person.
- Refocus the meeting on the original topic after the disruptive behavior has stopped.

Often people do not realize how their behavior is negatively influencing the other participants or the group process. The leader's goal is to preserve everyone's self-esteem while, at the same time, stopping the disruptive behavior. If continual efforts in the meeting fail, it is advisable to discuss recurring behavior privately with the person involved rather than to continue to confront the person (even indirectly) during the meeting.

Managing Diversity

Diversity is essential to a group and it is one of the primary values of ethics committees. Diversity increases energy and often leads to greater innovation. People learn to understand and respect each other more fully. Creative ideas flow more freely in such an environment and committees reach higher quality decisions when they can allow and explore divergent input. Effective diversity has substance to it. It arises because people have different facts or experiences, or because people interpret data differently. Getting several points of view on an issue is always valuable. Each person has the ability to see the topic from a different angle. An effective leader needs to be able to encourage this diversity while maintaining positive results. As with other group leadership skills, managing diversity is a careful balancing act between soliciting divergent views and preventing destructive conflict.

If different points of view are not requested, they are frequently not given. The leader needs to solicit diversity of information and views and should start the meeting by encouraging everyone to express his or her honest opinion. The leader may also specifically ask for different points of view or question the assumptions that everyone appears to be using. In a group in which there is little disagreement or diversity, it may be useful to appoint someone as a devil's advocate, one who tries to make the case for a deliberately different view of the issue.

When diversity is encouraged, some ideas will not be accepted. People sometimes become defensive when their ideas are criticized or rejected. They interpret this as a criticism or rejection of themselves. With strong personal involvement, members lose their objectivity about their own contributions. Unless some steps are taken, group members may be prone to associate an idea too closely with the originator himself. In order to prevent this, everyone should refrain from referring to an idea as "Jim's" or "Mary's" idea. Instead, they should refer to it as "an alternative" or "the idea." An idea should always be weighed on its merit, of course, not on its source.

If diversity leads to substantive conflict (for example, if the group becomes polarized), then the leader faces a difficult challenge. If not handled carefully, the conflict can develop into personal anger or animosity and can significantly interfere with all the committee's workings. When substantive disagreement is substantial, the leader would be well advised to articulate carefully the areas of common agreement.

Focusing on agreement puts things into perspective, for the areas of disagreement are usually small in comparison to the areas of agreement. Then, the points of disagreement and their causes should be carefully defined. This will couch the disagreement in more objective terms, taking it from the realm of feelings and making it appear more manageable. Finally, the entire topic may need to be tabled until later, when people will be less "invested" in the disagreement itself. When substantial disagreements arise, members may lose interest in the main thrust of the discussions and fix on the disagreement. By moving the group either back to the ideas that were being discussed before the disagreement arose or on to the next set of ideas, the flow of the meeting can be regained.

Trust, respect, and productivity are the hallmarks of a skilled group leader. The better the leadership, the more efficiently and effectively a group works. Becoming a good leader takes time, but if all members of the committee spend some time thinking about group process they will then be aware of how each member can contribute to making the committee work better. It is unreasonable to expect the leader to behave responsibly and conscientiously, while assuming that the committee members may behave unconsciously and erratically. The leader must take responsibility for guiding the process, but all committee members should be aware of their own responsibilities and should work to become productive members of the group and to effectively contribute to the group process.

Note

1. Group Action is a training system designed by Zenger Miller, management training consultant, Cupertino, CA

Appendix E

Evaluation Questions

Committee evaluation forms should be devised to obtain as much information as possible without taxing the limited time of the members. A questionnaire should not be very long if it includes many open-ended questions. Because most open-ended questions require the respondent to think about and articulate an individual answer, more than 8 to 10 questions are likely to cause the respondents to become impatient with the form. When preparing a questionnaire, consider whether you yourself could answer the questions without investing a substantial amount of time and thought. It is unfortunate, but questions must be relatively easy to answer—in one or two sentences—or people will generally not answer them. Although they may have much to say on a topic, many people do not frequently express their opinions in writing and they often find it difficult to do so when asked. Remember also that yes-or-no questions may provide too little information. Thus, questions should be neither too simple nor too complex.

Think about what kind of information will be most helpful to the committee and orient the questions to those areas. For example, is the committee interested in knowing what effect being on the committee has on the person? In how the committee's work is perceived? In whether or not the committee structures are appropriate? In general, it is best to put questions that are easier to answer at the beginning and the more demanding questions at the end. To the greatest extent possible, questionnaires should be anonymous (although this may sometimes be difficult to achieve).

These questions are intended only as suggestions. Other questions may be even more appropriate to a committee's own situation.

- How long have you been a member of the committee?
- Have you attended more than three-fourths of the meetings during that time?
- If not, why not? (time conflicts, attendance not necessary to fulfill responsibilities, other)
- Have you ever served on a subcommittee?
- Did the orientation provided when you joined the committee give you an adequate initial background?
- While you have been a member of the committee, what reading or study on bioethics issues have you done in addition to that specifically required by membership?
- Does being on the committee require you to do more than attend meetings?
- Do you personally subscribe to bioethics journals (for example, *Hastings Center Report* or *Law, Medicine and Health Care*)?

- What have been the committee's most important achievements during the time you were on the committee? During the past year?
- What are the committee's biggest problems?
- What is your opinion of the committee's case reviews?
- If you were a patient, would you be comfortable having the committee review your case without your knowledge?
- Do you think the committee should concentrate on a single area rather than trying to provide education, to write policies, and to conduct case review? If so, on which area should it concentrate?
- Do you participate in educational offerings made by the committee?
- Do you think the committee's work is effective?
- Do you think the committee's work is necessary?
- Would you recommend membership on the committee to those with whom you work? To friends in the hospital?
- Do you believe that everyone on the committee has an equal voice (as opposed to the group being dominated by a few individuals)?
- Do you believe that the physicians tend to dominate committee decisions?
- If your committee has an ethicist as a member, do you find that helpful? Does the viewpoint of the ethicist tend to dominate decisions?
- If your committee has an attorney as a member, do you find that helpful? Does the attorney tend to dominate decisions?
- Do you know more about ethical issues in health care after being on the committee?
- After completing a term on the committee, would you apply for membership again at a later time?
- Does being a member of the committee affect your work in any way? How?
- Does membership on the committee give you a better understanding of the problems faced by other health care providers (physicians, nurses, social workers, administrators, pastoral care givers)?
- Does membership on the committee give you a better understanding of the strengths possessed by other health care providers (physicians, nurses, social workers, administrators, pastoral care givers)?
- Do you receive enough education and educational guidance and opportunities to feel competent to contribute to the committee's work?
- Do you ever act as an informal educator among your colleagues as a result of your membership on the committee?
- Do the people with whom you work know that you are a member of the ethics committee?

- Do they perceive you as a resource for them on ethical questions?
- Is the committee too large? Too small?
- Does it meet often enough to carry out its work?
- Are the meetings long enough to complete scheduled business?

- Are the meetings conducted in an efficient manner?
- In your opinion, what is the committee's purpose?
- Do you believe the committee achieved its goals during the past year?
- What single thing would you change about the committee if you could?

Appendix **F**

Case Studies and Analyses

This appendix includes several typical cases, the first one of which is analyzed by four persons who are members of ethics committees. Although each of the reviewers comes to the same general conclusion, it is worth noting that, as is typical, each focuses her review on different details of the case. In addition, all four insist upon further information. This, too, is typical of case reviews. The information that is offered is almost never sufficient. Additional information is sometimes readily available from those presenting the case, but at other times committee members ask questions that no one involved in the case has thought to ask. Although waiting may be inconvenient, frequently a recommendation should be delayed while further information is gathered. In many, and perhaps most, cases for which adequate information is provided committee members are likely to agree about a recommendation. The second and third case studies do not include analyses. Committees may wish to use these to develop their own skills in case review.

Case Study 1: Mrs. J

Mrs. J is a 55-year-old woman. She was previously an accountant but is now retired because of disability. She was widowed fifteen years ago and has not remarried. She has one married, adult daughter, age 35. Mrs. J has a long history of rheumatic heart disease. Her current admission was for mitral valve replacement surgery. Multiple complications ensued during surgery, including a right ventricular tear of the heart, bleeding requiring multiple blood transfusions, and prolonged time on the cardiac bypass pump. Her postsurgery course has been difficult. She has adult respiratory distress syndrome and continues to be respirator dependent seven weeks after surgery. She has not tolerated attempts to wean her from the ventilator; her body systems seem to be very delicately balanced. She is quickly fatigued but is occasionally able to sit in a chair for meals.

Her physicians are guardedly optimistic about her chances for recovery. They believe that she can be weaned from the respirator but that this will take at least several more months. Even if this occurs, they are uncertain about how much physical activity she will regain. It is possible that she will continue to be confined to bed for much of the time.

During the past week, she has experienced two cardiac arrests. She responded quickly after the first one with no chest compressions. The next day, she talked with her minister and then asked her physicians not to resuscitate her should she experience cardiac arrest again. The physicians believe that this request is premature given the prognosis. Her daughter was completely opposed to a do-not-resuscitate (DNR) order. Mrs. J withdrew her request. At the time of the second cardiac arrest, however, Mrs. J asked the nurse to let her die; the nurse called for resuscitation, which was achieved with only a few chest compressions.

Three days have passed since the second arrest. Mrs. J has again requested that her physician write a DNR order for her. She is rested and alert; there is no question of incompetence. The physicians have discussed their belief that she can be weaned from the ventilator and that, although she will probably not recover complete physical function, she will continue to have some ability to move about and to retain full mental capacity. The physicians and the daughter continue to be opposed to the request for a DNR order. Other care givers have mixed feelings and opinions.

Mrs. J: Analysis A

My first reaction to the facts presented is reluctance to accept the idea of a DNR order for someone so young and for whom the prognosis is the possibility of continued survival with full mental capacity. There is a tendency in situations like this to question the patient's competence but, we are told, there is no question of incompetence. I want to know more. What is Mrs. J's understanding of her prognosis? What other persons are part of her life besides her daughter? Once Mrs. J went home, what would her circumstances be? Who would take care of her? Who would she talk to? It is appropriate to consider a person's right to make her own decision as a first principle, but this does not mean we need to accept immediately her perception of her life. We need at least to explore the possibility that the perception is inaccurate, or, if accurate, that it is susceptible to change.

On the other hand, we need to know more about what is behind the physicians' and the daughter's opposition to a DNR order. Are the physicians truly convinced the prognosis is good enough to justify their position? Is the daughter really paying attention to her mother's interests or is she acting out of guilt for past neglect? How much responsibility is she planning to take once her mother is out of the hospital?

Before viewing this situation as an ethical dilemma, I would want to know if social services has been involved with this family. Has someone spent time with Mrs. J exploring her feelings and her fears? Is Mrs. J aware of the resources that might be available? Have her friends been mobilized as a support system? What about the minister to whom Mrs. J spoke? Can her church be more helpful to her? Also, has the daughter had an opportunity to explore her feelings about her mother's illness?

More information is needed from the physicians. How much longer can Mrs. J expect to live? Will further arrests decrease the chance of her retaining full mental capacity?

What about the other care givers? What is the source of their mixed feelings? Do they think the physicians are unduly optimistic? Has their observation of the mother-daughter relationship made them skeptical about the support Mrs. J would receive once out of the hospital? The input of nurses and other care givers can add much to the ethics committee's understanding of the situation.

What about Mrs. J's state of mind? She may be competent, but is it possible that she has a treatable depression? Is she willing to talk to a clinical social worker, psychiatrist, or other mental health professional? It might be interesting to explore why she has not asked to be taken off the ventilator.

The point of all these questions is that a situation should not be labeled an ethical dilemma until all the facts are known and other approaches have been explored. Then and only then should we frame the situation as an ethical dilemma, placing Mrs. J's autonomy in opposition to the beneficence of the physicians and of the daughter. If none of the alternative approaches has been productive and this conflict turns out to be real, then Mrs. J's autonomy must prevail. In my view, the autonomy of a competent person takes precedence over the beneficence of care givers as an ethical principle. In addition, our legal system makes autonomy a central value and past court cases indicate that Mrs. J would have her right to decide on a DNR order vindicated were she to take her case to court.

Mrs. J: Analysis B

On the surface, this case concerns a competent patient who understands the implications of her decision requesting that a standard form of treatment (CPR) be foregone. If a competent, adult patient always has a right to refuse any treatment, including life-prolonging treatment, then Mrs. J's request should be honored by her physicians and respected by her daughter, even if they do not agree with her choice. Clearly, this is a case in which patient autonomy comes into conflict with physician beneficence. Autonomy is frequently stated to be the primary value in such a conflict. Yet, in this case, one draws back from that simple response in the face of two considerations.

First, the patient and her daughter are in direct conflict on what care is appropriate. If patient and family are united in their preferences for nontreatment, it is often easier to accept the primacy of their position. Because both the patient and the family must live (or die) with the consequences of foregoing life-prolonging treatment, the decision involves each person's sense of self. Although Mrs. J is an individual, she is not an individual who lives without connections to others. The ties between parent and child run deep, and the effects of those ties are often not consciously understood. The division in this case may suggest that the mother, but not the daughter, is able to accept the mother's death, and that the daughter's feelings are being reinforced by her alliance with the physicians. Although one might be concerned about legal implications of foregoing treatment when the daughter opposes it, that concern clearly has no strong ethical basis considering the deference customarily paid to patient autonomy. There is, however, an ethical basis for being concerned with the daughter's alienation from her mother's wishes. One needs to know something more about the daughter before concluding that her wishes should be entirely ignored. For example, what kind of relationship has she had with her mother? Is her unwillingness to see her mother die based on her own need for her mother to live or on her knowledge of her mother's characteristic ways of thinking and feeling?

The second difficulty is in the information that is available to us. Mrs. J's prognosis is not extremely good, but she appears neither to be terminally ill nor to be facing imminent death. Foregoing life-saving treatment in the absence of these conditions needs to be looked at carefully. Mrs. J has apparently been disabled for some time (she is retired because of disability), but we are unsure of her mode of living prior to this operation. If her recovery is maximal, will she be worse than she was previously? In addition, we do not know precisely why she does not want resuscitation. Is it that she believes her quality of life will be too low to offer sufficient rewards? Is she concerned about how she will be able to care for herself? Are there financial concerns? Are there psychological concerns about loss of independence or being a burden on her daughter? Without this information, it is difficult to assess her full understanding of her situation. She may be competent and she may understand the implications of her wish not to be resuscitated. Nevertheless, when a patient's death is the result of a decision to refuse treatment and death is not inevitable, those who must preside over that death have both a professional obligation and a human obligation to understand why the patient is making that choice.

Given that information about these two important considerations is missing, a decision to forego

CPR ought to be postponed, at least for a brief period, while acknowledging to Mrs. J that the physicians have some uncertainties that need to be pursued before they write the DNR order. That is, the physicians should not be pressing for a different decision. Their duty, having provided their best judgment to her, is to support her wishes. Since death is permanent, however, the obligation of beneficence requires them to make sure that her decision is based on an appropriate view of reality. Whoever has the ability to talk with this family (priest, nurse, social worker, physician, psychotherapist) needs to do so in order to elicit the missing information.

The reasons both for the mother's wish to forego CPR and for the daughter's wish that she receive CPR should be sought. If the daughter does not provide some relevant information that would affect one's assessment of Mrs. J's character (for example, that she is prone to severe depressive bouts), and if it is clear that Mrs. J's preferences are not based on unrealistic or inappropriate fears (for example, that she will be a burden to her daughter, whereas either her care could be accommodated by someone other than the daughter or the daughter genuinely needs her mother and the mother's death would thus be a greater burden than her illness), then the DNR order should be written, even if the physicians and the daughter disapprove. If the DNR order is to be written, every effort should be made to help the daughter understand why her mother chooses this route and accept her mother's decision to forego CPR. The important disagreement, assuming that the medical information about prognosis is correct and that Mrs. J understands what it means for her, is between the mother and daughter, not between the mother and the physicians. Mrs. J's refusal of CPR should be honored if she judges, upon reflection, that the quality of life that will be available to her is not acceptable and if her judgment appears, to a neutral observer, to be consistent with actual facts.

Postscript: One additional issue in this case deserves mention. The physicians' disagreement with the patient is, from my perspective, significantly strengthened by the fact that the daughter shares this disagreement. One might question how the daughter came to be informed of the patient's request. In many such situations, physicians who disagree with a patient's assessment of the appropriate action go to the family and request their help in "getting the patient to see reason" (or some such phrase). It should be noted that a patient's request for a DNR order, like all other information about the patient, falls under an obligation of confidentiality. The information should not be revealed to others, including family members, without the specific consent of the patient (as long as the patient is competent; when he or she is incompetent, other standards of judgment need to be applied). If the information was revealed to the daughter without the patient's consent, then Mrs. J's autonomy has already been significantly diminished. Under such circumstances, patients may well insist upon asserting *their* will against that of the physician, if only to demonstrate that they are still in charge of their lives (or deaths).

Mrs. J: Analysis C

The case of Mrs. J may not, at first glance, seem to provide much discussion or deliberation for an ethics committee. Certainly it does not evoke the same strong polarized discussion as does a case centering on the issue of feeding. Nor is it likely to bring out the questions and concerns often associated with discontinuing a ventilator from a competent patient. Yet the case is one that should sound very familiar to doctors, nurses, and other health care professionals working with critically ill patients. It is a good example of one of the most frequent conflicts of values seen in health care today: autonomy versus beneficence. The very fact that it does not cause strong emotional reactions should cause us to examine more "everyday" cases for the presence of value conflicts. In order to evaluate Mrs. J's case, I would look first at the medical facts, then explore the values at stake, examine all possible options, and finally recommend an option that supported the values.

The medical facts of Mrs. J's case are relatively straightforward. Mrs. J is currently ventilator-dependent due to compromised respiratory-circulatory status. Although attempts to this point to wean Mrs. J have been unsuccessful, her physicians do believe that she can eventually be weaned. Her prognosis for recovery from adult respiratory distress syndrome (ARDS) is good although her long-range prognosis is fair. That is, she most likely will have limited mobility and will remain a chronically ill patient.

Although the prognosis for recovery from ARDS is good, currently Mrs. J is unstable as reflected by two cardiac arrests experienced in the last week. Although the reasons for the arrests are not specifically stated, one might assume they are related to the "failing" heart.

There are other facts that are important to consider in Mrs. J's case. First of all, she is described as rested and alert. It is made clear that there is no question of incompetence. The implication, of course, is that Mrs. J is capable of consenting to, refusing to consent to, or withdrawing consent for any medical procedures during her hospitalization. She is the primary decision maker in regard to her care. Although Mrs. J is responsible for her decisions, she is in interaction with others regarding those decisions. Her adult daughter is available, as is a minister. We have no other information regarding Mrs. J, such as her life style prior to this hospitalization or her financial status, points that might be explored.

As stated previously, the values in conflict here are fairly obvious. The physicians' value of beneficence (doing good for the patient) is very strong. This patient is not terminally ill and although her situation is currently unstable, the prognosis for recovery from ARDS is good. CPR, in their opinion, would certainly benefit the patient, as has already been demonstrated twice. The conflict arises when we realize that Mrs. J is requesting that no resuscitation efforts be instituted. The value here is patient autonomy, the right to decide one's own course of treatment. We must consider which of these values—beneficence or autonomy—takes priority.

Most of the literature in bioethics supports patient autonomy as the priority value. This is not a commentary on the physicians' values being less worthwhile, only a recognition that the right to self-determination is one that is clearly supported in this country. Certainly there are questions that must be asked. Autonomy implies more than simply making the decision for one's self. It implies understanding the consequences of that decision and having the proper information to arrive at that decision.

What are the possible options in Mrs. J's situation? First, the physicians could continue to treat Mrs. J aggressively with full resuscitation efforts. Although this would certainly be understandable in light of the physicians' beliefs that resuscitation will benefit Mrs. J, it would certainly not support patient autonomy. Second, the physician could accept Mrs. J's wishes and write a do-not-resuscitate order on her chart. While obviously supporting Mrs. J's desires, this course may present some problems. Does she indeed understand the nature of her decision? What will be her daughter's response? In light of these questions, I think the third option would be to have a discussion with all the involved parties (that is, Mrs. J, her physicians, her daughter, and the other health care professionals involved). Foremost, it must be determined that Mrs. J does understand that CPR will benefit her and perhaps allow the physicians time to bring her to a more comfortable physical state. Second, Mrs. J must clearly understand the consequences of refusing CPR. If her daughter is present, Mrs. J can listen to her concerns and consider these along with the medical information as she makes her decision. If Mrs. J

remains firm in her request not to be resuscitated, I believe the hospital and the physicians are obligated to follow her wishes. If the physicians feel strongly that this is inappropriate, they can certainly turn Mrs. J's care over to another physician.

This case is important because of its seemingly benign nature. All too often when a patient is not terminally ill and CPR may obviously benefit the patient, health care professionals insist on "doing everything." Frequently, patient requests are overridden because of concerns regarding depression and lack of understanding. Health care professionals, who often describe themselves as patient advocates, act clearly in ways that place the patient as an outsider in his or her own care.

What would be the role of a bioethics committee in Mrs. J's case? Because of the obvious disagreement between Mrs J. and her daughter and physicians, the bioethics committee may become involved. The committee's role, though, should be to promote the type of discussion described above with Mrs. J. There is a temptation here for the committee to step in and "solve" the problem, but they have neither the authority nor the right to do that. It could serve to lessen Mrs. J's autonomy even more. The committee's role should be to explore the issues with those involved, to help them to clarify the dilemma, to promote the recognition of values, and to support the efforts of all those involved as they accept Mrs. J.'s direction of the course of her care.

Mrs. J: Analysis D

Some unanswered questions in this case should be addressed before I would be bold enough to render an opinion. For example, some medical facts are unclear. Is Mrs. J having cardiac or respiratory arrests? What is the suspected cause? Is the situation expected to change?

My main concerns have to do with Mrs. J's state of mind. Why is she so opposed to a resuscitation effort? Does the procedure itself repel her? Is she discouraged at the prospect of several more months on the ventilator? Is it the prospect of limited physical capacity, predicted by the doctors to be her lot even if she is weaned from the ventilator, that bothers her? In short, is she as clear as possible about her situation and is she able to give a truly informed refusal of treatment? Might she change her mind if she progressed to the point where she felt better?

One of the things that a health professional rarely knows about a patient (unless they have had a long-standing relationship) is how the person's behavior as a patient compares with his or her usual patterns of thinking and acting. On one hand, Mrs. J may be a woman who has considerable zest for living but is in a temporary slump because of her current health crisis. If so, she may need coaxing to get through these rough weeks so that she may look with more optimism to the future.

On the other hand, she may in recent years have become discouraged at the state of her health and set some personal limits to what she is willing to endure from now on. If she feels that the limited existence predicted by her physicians would be too burdensome for her, she may be unwilling to go through several more months on a ventilator, with occasional cardiac resuscitations, to get to that ultimate unhappy point.

Who is likely to know Mrs. J well enough to answer these questions? Her daughter may be able to; however, for various reasons, she may not. The priest mentioned may know her well, or he may know of someone who does. Mrs. J. does not appear to be saying, "Let me die *now*." If she were, she could ask that the ventilator be removed; instead she is asking that she not be revived if her heart stops. It is necessary to be as clear as possible about why she feels this way. The answer to that question should lead to more appropriate next steps.

Whatever her state of mind, Mrs. J is probably not comfortable with the fact that no one seems to understand her point of view. It may be that she subconsciously wants resistance from those around her so that she is assured of continued treatment (some patients are like this), but she could be genuinely distressed that she is fighting the battle alone. Unfortunately, such feelings are common with patients, especially very sick ones. In our zeal to do well by them medically, we can forget that they need attention spiritually and emotionally. Mrs. J. will be fortunate if someone can be found who is as interested in listening to her feelings as in compressing her heart. This should be done as openly and carefully as possible, without preconceived notions about what she is saying or "should" be saying. She may or may not decide to request a DNR order. Her final decision is less important than the opportunity she has to make it.

Case Study 2: JL

JL is a 36-year-old male admitted to the hospital through the emergency department with suspected acquired immune deficiency syndrome (AIDS). Presenting symptoms included severe dehydration and wasting due to prolonged anorexia and diarrhea. Physical examination revealed diffused lymphadenopathy and extensive purplish nodules on his extremities and trunk. The patient also complained of shortness of breath and persistent cough. His personal history revealed JL to be a sexually active homosexual male, living with his lover for three years. Diagnostic studies revealed the lesions to be Kaposi's sarcoma and chest X ray confirmed pneumocystis carinii pneumonia. Laboratory studies revealed cytomegalovirus and HTLV-III antibodies. JL was placed in isolation and treatment for the opportunistic infections was begun. The clinical picture suggested an advanced state of AIDS.

JL's condition deteriorated over three weeks, and he was transferred to ICU. Weight loss, fever, and diarrhea continued as well as increasing respiratory difficulty. Bilateral lung consolidation finally resulted in intubation and mechanical ventilation. The Kaposi's sarcoma continued to spread and had become inflamed, oozing a purulent discharge. Hypertension resulted in vasopressor therapy. JL had initially been coherent and alert, but as his condition deteriorated, he was no longer able to communicate with the staff.

As his prognosis worsened, the health care team discussed his plan of care. The physicians reported that the rapid deterioration and failure to respond to treatment suggested little hope. Further aggressive treatment appeared futile.

Help was sought from JL's family. His mother and father have had difficulty in dealing with their son's illness, especially because they had not known of his homosexuality until this hospitalization. Although they actively supported JL while he was able to communicate, since his deterioration they have requested that no aggressive treatment be initiated, including CPR. This is in direct opposition to what JL's lover has requested. Stating that he and JL discussed this quite openly, his lover has asked that *everything* be done. "JL asked me not to let them give up trying," he said. He insists that JL remain a full code and that aggressive treatment continue.

The staff members have mixed emotions regarding the extent of treatment. Although they have willingly cared for JL, they are unsure about exposing themselves to the risk of contracting AIDS through CPR in light of the questionable benefit of CPR to JL. As a result of these questions, staff nurses have asked that the ethics committee consult with them on the case.

Case Study 3: Mildred Montgomery

In 1979, Mildred Montgomery, an 84-year-old woman suffering from increased confusion, was admitted to a nursing home. The patient had never married. Her three sisters, to whom she was close, had died. Her only living relative was a nephew, who was appointed her guardian just prior to her nursing home admission.

Over the next three years, her condition deteriorated to the point where she was described by physicians as being "severely demented." The patient did not respond to verbal stimuli. She followed movements with her eyes; used her hands to scratch herself; and was able to move her head, neck, arms, and hands voluntarily. A nurse reported that the patient smiled when she was massaged or her hair was combed, and moaned when she was fed. Severe contractions of her lower legs kept her in a semifetal position. She developed necrotic ulcers on her left foot as a complication of diabetes.

In 1982, a nasogastric tube was placed in the patient because she was no longer able to take suffi-cient food and liquids by mouth. Several months later, the nephew requested that the nasogastric feeding be discontinued and the patient be kept comfortable until she died. The physician has requested a meeting with the nursing home ethics committee, with respect to whether nasogastric feeding is "ordinary" or "extraordinary" treatment.

References

Abrams, N., and Buckner, M. D. *Medical Ethics: A Clinical Textbook and Reference for the Health Care Professions.* Cambridge, MA: MIT Press, 1983, pp. 589-640.

Levine, C., and Veatch, R. M. *Cases in Bioethics.* Hastings-on-Hudson, NY: Hastings Center, 1982.

Appendix **G**

Religion and Health Care Ethics

Ethics committees may find that in some situations the patient's and family's religious values contribute to disagreements about what kind of treatment is acceptable. This appendix does not attempt an exhaustive survey of organized religions' positions on health care issues. It does, however, try to alert ethics committee members to some issues that may arise. *The Encyclopedia of Bioethics*[1] offers discussions of the views of many different religious groups, including a number not included in this summary.

Roman Catholic Teachings on Specific Forms of Medical Care

Abortion

The Roman Catholic church has always taken a very strict view about the impermissibility of abortion and it has reiterated that view frequently in recent years. The teaching is that no *direct* killing of an innocent person is ever permitted. *Indirect* abortion (in which the death of the fetus is a foreseen but unintended side effect) is permitted for sufficient reasons. The two most often used examples of indirect abortion are the removal of a cancerous uterus when the woman is pregnant and the removal of a portion of the fallopian tube containing an ectopic pregnancy.

Contraception, Sterilization, and Reproduction

The church's official position is that all methods of artificial birth control are morally wrong. Contraception is held to be morally wrong because it divorces the unitive function of the marital act from the procreative function. Extraordinary forms of reproduction (artificial insemination, in vitro fertilization, and, probably by extension, surrogacy and embryo transfer) are also considered wrong, but for the reverse reason. In these instances, the procreative function is divorced from the unitive function.

Some contemporary theologians argue that artificial insemination by the husband should be permitted because the couple are not separating the unitive and procreative functions by choice. In vitro fertilization is generally disapproved even when the husband's sperm is used because it totally separates the unitive and procreative functions, although some theologians find it acceptable because its intention is to create new life. However, extraordinary forms of reproduction are generally frowned upon, not only for

more traditional reasons, but because they could have a negative effect on the child and also on society in the long run.

Brain Death

In 1957, Pope Pius XII, in his address to an International Congress of Anesthesiologists, took the position that the time when death occurs is beyond the competency of the church or of theology and belongs to medical science.

Suicide, Euthanasia, and the Prolongation of Life

Roman Catholic moral teaching has consistently opposed suicide and euthanasia (mercy killing) on the grounds that an individual person exercises stewardship, not full dominion, over his or her life. References are frequently made to natural law arguments, to scriptural arguments, and to the evil consequences that would flow from euthanasia. However, pain medication can be given to dying persons, even though these drugs may have an indirect effect of hastening that person's death.

Clearly distinct from suicide and active euthanasia is the teaching that one does not have to use "extraordinary means" to preserve human life. The terms *ordinary* and *extraordinary* have been used in the past to refer to treatments that were or were not morally obligatory with respect to prolonging life. Because these terms are often unclear, the Vatican Congregation for the Doctrine of the Faith suggested, in 1980, that the words "proportionate" and "disproportionate" might be an improvement. Both of these pairs of words are meant to apply to the effect of the treatment on the patient, rather than to anything intrinsic to the treatment itself. The church has always taught that if a medical intervention either imposes too great a hardship on the patient or offers no reasonable hope of benefit, it is considered disproportionate and is therefore not morally required.

Other Issues

There are numerous other areas of ethical concern to those who receive health care. Among them are such issues as justice, care for the poor, privacy, truth-telling, confidentiality, organ transplants, genetics, experimentation, the treatment of rape victims, and the treatment of newborns with disabilities. For a more thorough discussion of these issues, the reader is referred to the books by Ashley and O'Rourke and by McCormick, listed at the end of this appendix. In addition, *Ethical and Religious Directives for Catholic Health Facilities* was published in pamphlet form by the American bishops to give direction to Catholic health care institutions. It mentions the following topics: abortion, treatment of hemorrhage during pregnancy, caesarean section, intrauterine pregnancy, hysterectomy, sterilization, artificial insemination, masturbation for seminal analysis, experimentation, "mercy killing," giving medications for pain, organ transplants, postmortem examinations, ghost surgery, and the cremation of a fetus or a part of the body.

Protestant Perspectives on Specific Forms of Medical Care

Because Protestantism is characterized by individual insight and individual freedom of thought, the many Protestant denominations are less likely than the Roman Catholic church to have a delineated position on specific health care issues. In some cases, however, there are guidelines that are not intended to be binding upon the members. In even fewer cases, there are strict positions. In general, Protestant views on health care stress "concern for the personal integrity of the patient and ways to promote his spiritual and psychological growth."[2] The positions listed below are drawn from several sources and are stated generally. More detailed information is available in *Religious Aspects of Medical Care* (Catholic Hospital Association, 1975), a short book listing the views of forty different religious groups on specific issues in health care.

Abortion, Contraception, and Reproduction

Because abortion has provoked so much dispute within American society, many denominations have taken specific positions on the practice. Some approve therapeutic abortions (that is, to protect the mother's life or health), but not elective abortions. Episcopalians, the Assembly of God, Jehovah's Witnesses, Latter Day Saints, American Lutherans, and Wisconsin Evangelical Lutherans all oppose elective abortion.

Latter Day Saints and Wisconsin Evangelical Lutherans oppose contraception, and Jehovah's Witnesses discourage contraception and oppose sterilization.

American Lutherans and Wisconsin Evangelical Lutherans oppose the use of artificial insemination by donor (AID) other than spouse, while Jehovah's Witnesses disapprove of any form of artificial insemination, as well as any genetics/eugenics practices. Presbyterians do not oppose AID or surrogate mother

practices, but suggest that further study be given to determine the ethical, psychological, and legal ramifications of these practices. They are less comfortable with eugenics practices intended to develop "superior" human beings.

Transplantation

American Lutherans do not acknowledge a duty to donate body parts. Jehovah's Witnesses regard donating and receiving body organs for transplantation as a matter of individual conscience. Christian Scientists, who generally eschew standard medical care, would be unlikely to find transplantation acceptable.

Foregoing Life-Prolonging Treatment

Most denominations prohibit active euthanasia and generally accept refusing or withholding treatment when death is inevitable or, in some cases, when continued life is very burdensome either for the patient or for the patient's family. The Presbyterian statement strongly urges individuals to take care in considering the question of refusing treatment and to provide instructions (such as a living will) indicating personal preferences. The Presbyterian policy statement also suggests a stronger view about the wisdom of providing treatment for permanently unconscious patients by stating that "it is indeed idolatrous to try to keep a person's body alive no matter how empty that life may be. . . . Real life comes from beyond bodily function."[3]

Blood Transfusions

Jehovah's Witnesses forbid all blood transfusions as a violation of scriptural command.

Jewish Perspectives on Specific Forms of Medical Care

Because there is no single central authority for Judaism (as there is in Catholicism) and because answers depend upon interpretation from many different sources over time, two (or more) rabbis may disagree about the proper answer to a question. As a result, Jewish thought frequently does not provide single, undisputed answers to new topics such as those raised in medical ethics.

In addition, it is difficult to state "the Jewish position" because Judaism is divided into three subgroups: Orthodox, Conservative, and Reform. Orthodox Jews believe that Jewish law must be interpreted literally, unchanging throughout the ages. Conservative Jews believe that the law is binding upon them, but the ways of responding to the law can be adapted to meet the contemporary context. Reform Jews, the most liberal, see the law as nonbinding, but providing guidance in making individual decisions. Because each group's perspective on the meaning of the law differs, their rabbinic interpretations may also differ. The force of those rabbinic responsa (or interpretations) also differs. Orthodox and Conservative Jews are expected to act in accordance with the responsa. Reform Jews look at responsa, as they look at all the law, as guidance for individual decision making.

In this discussion of specific health care issues, the reader should keep in mind that many Jews do not identify themselves with either the Orthodox, Conservative, or Reform branches, but rather see themselves as ethnic, secular Jews. Furthermore, the positions described are more likely to correspond to the views of Orthodox or Conservative Jews rather than those of Reform Jews.

Judaism does not allow for individualistic "ownership of body" claims. With respect to health care, Jews have an obligation to care for their health and, if they are ill, they have a duty to seek medical care. The object of medical care should be to preserve life. Jewish physicians have a corresponding duty to provide medical care and to preserve life.

Abortion

Jewish thought holds that a fetus is not a person until it is born (specifically, until its head emerges). Thus, there is no question about the fetus being a person from conception and abortion being thereby forbidden. However, despite the fetus's lack of personhood, abortion is discouraged and sometimes prohibited because the fetus has the potential for personhood and thus is not a morally neutral object. Also, as noted above, there is a belief that the body belongs to God, not to the person, and therefore abortion justified by women's claims of ownership of their bodies is not acceptable. Rosner cites four bases for the general prohibition on abortion: the command to multiply and be fruitful, the potential or partial person status of the fetus, the prohibition on self-injury (by and/or to the woman), and the danger to the woman.[4]

Decisions about the acceptability of abortion fall for the most part solely upon questions of the effect upon the mother. When her life or health is threatened, abortion is clearly permissible and may even be required. When the question is based upon the nature of the fetus's life (that is, when there are genetic or developmental abnormalities), some author-

ities say that even though the fetus is not a person, the fetus's health should be considered independently. This might justify abortion for severe anomalies, but the commentators are clearly concerned that this permission not be used lightly. Similarly, there is little support for abortion because of a claim of rape, except insofar as the woman's health (physical and mental) is at risk from the pregnancy. Abortion on demand is not acceptable.

Contraception

Because of God's command to be fruitful and multiply, contraception is generally discouraged. The command, however, is to men, rather than to women and, as a result, female contraception is more acceptable. The use of condoms, abstinence, and *coitus interruptus* are forbidden in all instances. Non-Orthodox Jews (Conservative, Reform) are much more liberal about the use of contraception, except that demographic concerns sometimes temper that judgment. Because of the loss of so many Jews in the Holocaust, the high incidence of intermarriage, and the low birth rate of Jewish couples, pressures continue among all Jewish groups against the use of contraception.

Sterilization and Reproduction

Sterilization of males is generally prohibited by both the Orthodox and non-Orthodox, unless it is a matter of saving life or health. It is more acceptable for women but, in the absence of a threat to life or health, she should already have given birth to at least two children.

Most rabbis find artificial insemination by husband (AIH) acceptable as a way of complying with the command to have children. Twenty years ago, most commentators found artificial insemination by donor (AID) to be an unacceptable method of overcoming infertility. They were concerned, in particular, with AID as a form of adultery (with the prospect of future incest, the child not knowing its genetic father) and with the implied threat to basic values (home, marriage, family ties). Nevertheless, many rabbis today find AID acceptable, not the least because of the need to encourage reproduction among a Jewish population with a declining birth rate.

The practice of surrogate mothering (either through artificial insemination of a woman who will bear a child for the infertile couple or through the use of embryo transfer following AIH) has been declared by England's chief rabbi to be "a revolting degradation of maternity and an affront to human dignity."[5]

Definition of Death

Judaism traditionally defines death as the permanent cessation of breathing. Some commentators discuss the importance of the heartbeat but, generally, respiration is the critical factor. Because of this definition, there has been considerable hesitance in accepting heart transplantation, especially in its experimental stages. Attempts to redefine death in terms of brain function were not acceptable and there was considerable fear that the donor would not in fact be dead (by the Jewish definition) at the time the heart was removed. If the donor is not dead, then removing his or her heart is prohibited because "in order to save one life, one can never sacrifice another, in whatever lingering state of animation."[6] Although some conservative and reform rabbis have accepted EEG readings as a substitute criterion for death, most orthodox rabbis have not yet done so. Such acceptance is at least theoretically possible if a flat EEG is interpreted as another way of measuring the lost capacity for spontaneous respiration, rather than a substantively different definition of death.

Judaism permits organ transplantation whenever the donor is clearly dead according to Jewish law, or when a live donation is possible (kidney donation). Although Jewish law does not permit the desecration or mutilation of the body, organ donation is permitted if it is thereby possible to save another's life. This requirement for a life-saving procedure is liberally interpreted to include transplants not involving vital organs. Whenever an organ is donated, it is vitally important that the family consent to the donation. Dorff implies that the family consent is even more important than consent from the patient-donor because of the psychological effect that the donation will have upon them.[7]

Suicide, Euthanasia, and Prolongation of Life

Suicide is absolutely prohibited because one does not have the right to take a life that belongs to God. Suicide is strictly defined within the tradition, however. To be considered a suicide, a person must have stated his intention to take his own life and then must act in accordance with that intention.

Active euthanasia (commonly referred to as "mercy killing") is also prohibited because it constitutes murder. There is, furthermore, an extensive body of commentary that prohibits any action that will hasten death. The exception to this is that if a patient is moribund (facing imminent death) and death is expected to occur within three days, then it is possible to "remove impediments to the soul's departure."[8] Dorff, on the other hand, does not limit the withholding of treatment to the period when death is imminent, but rather claims that having a terminal illness alone constitutes justification.[9]

Jakobovitz adds that it is permissible to give analgesics to relieve pain, even though the dosage level risks hastening death. He maintains, however, that it is never permissible to withhold food, oxygen, or blood from the dying patient.[10]

Autopsy

The routine practice of autopsy is very controversial among Jews. It is generally discouraged, because it violates the prohibition against desecrating the body and that against profiting from the dead. For Orthodox and Conservative Jews, it is generally permitted only in those cases in which the life of an existing other person can be saved by the autopsy, there is a case of a hereditary disease and information can thereby be gained that will benefit others, the person gave consent while he or she was living, or it is needed for legal reasons. In the event of an autopsy, all organs of the body are to be returned to the body for burial. In those circumstances when a standard autopsy may not be performed, peritoneoscopy and needle biopsies are permitted.

Notes

1. Reich, W. T., ed. *Encyclopedia of Bioethics.* New York: Free Press, 1978.

2. Johnson, J. T. History of Protestant medical ethics. In: Reich, ed. *Encyclopedia of Bioethics.* 1978, p. 1368.

3. General Assembly (Presbyterian). *The Covenant of Life and the Caring Community.* Washington, DC: Office of the General Assembly, 1983, p. 24.

4. Rosner, F. *Modern Medicine and Jewish Law,* New York: Yeshiva University, 1972, pp.79-88.

5. Jakobovitz, I. *Jewish Medical Ethics,* 2nd ed. New York: Block Publishing Co., p. 265.

6. *Ibid.* p. 276.

7. Dorff, E. Choose life: A Jewish perspective on medical ethics. *University Papers.* 1985. 14(1):1-32.

8. Rosner, *Modern Medicine,* p. 121.

9. Dorff, "Choose life," p. 20.

10. Jakobovitz, *Jewish Medical Ethics,* p. 276.

References

Ashley, B. M., and O'Rourke, K. D. *Health Care Ethics,* 2nd ed. St. Louis: Catholic Health Association, 1982.

Catholic Hospital Association. *Religious Aspects of Medical Care.* St. Louis: CHA, 1975.

Curran, C. E. Roman Catholicism. In: Reich, W. T., ed. *Encyclopedia of Bioethics, 4 vols.* New York: Free Press, 1978, pp. 1522-34.

Dorff, E. Choose life: A Jewish perspective on medical ethics. *University Papers.* 1985, 14(1):1-32.

General Assembly (Presbyterian). *The Covenant of Life and the Caring Community.* Washington, DC: Office of the General Assembly, 1983.

Gershan, J. A. Judaic ethical beliefs and customs regarding death and dying. *Critical Care Nurse.* 1985. 5(1):32-4.

Gustafson, J. M. *Protestant and Roman Catholic Ethics.* Chicago: University of Chicago Press, 1978.

Jakobovitz, I. *Jewish Medical Ethics,* 2nd ed. New York: Block Publishing Co., 1975. (See, especially, pp. 251-294.)

Johnson, J. T. History of Protestant medical ethics. In: Reich, ed. *Encyclopedia of Bioethics,* New York: Free Press, 1978, pp. 1364-73.

Larue, G. A. *Euthanasia and Religion: A Survey of the Attitudes of World Religions to the Right-To-Die.* Los Angeles: Hemlock Society, 1985.

Marty, M. E., and Vaux, K. L., eds. *Health, Medicine, and the Faith Traditions.* Philadelphia: Fortress Press, 1982. (See, especially, Marty's "Introduction" and Vaux's "Topics at the Interface of Medicine and Theology" and "Theological Foundations of Medical Ethics.")

McCormick, R. A. *Health and Medicine in the Catholic Tradition.* New York: Crossroad Publishing Co., 1984.

Rosner, F. *Modern Medicine and Jewish Law.* New York: Yeshiva University, 1972.

United States Catholic Conference. *Ethical and Religious Directives for Catholic Health Facilities.* Washington, DC: United States Catholic Conference, 1977.

Vanderpool, H. Dominant health concerns in protestantism. In: Reich, W. T., ed. *Encyclopedia of Bioethics.* New York: Free Press, 1978, pp. 1373-8.

Vaux, K. L. *Biomedical Ethics.* New York: Harper and Row, 1974. (See, especially, "Protestantism," pp. 17-24.)

Annotated Bibliography

Books

Abrams, N., and Buckner, M. D. *Medical Ethics: A Clinical Textbook and Reference for the Health Care Professions*. Cambridge, MA: MIT Press, 1983.

This anthology includes an excellent and extensive selection of essays. The book has three major divisions: conceptual foundations, clinical ideals and behavior, and issues in clinical ethics. The appendixes include a series of case studies, the text of six important court decisions, and the text of a number of professional codes and statutes.

American Hospital Association. *Values in Conflict: Resolving Ethical Issues in Hospital Care*. Chicago: American Hospital Association, 1985.

This report is intended to be a guide for health care professionals responding to ethical dilemmas that arise in the hospital. It includes a discussion of the hospital's unique role in assuring good decision making, as well as practical guidelines.

Beauchamp, T., and Childress, J. *Principles of Biomedical Ethics*. 2nd ed. New York: Oxford University Press, 1983.

This clear, concise textbook explains basic ethical principles and shows how they are applied to such major issues in bioethics as informed consent, risk-benefit assessment, confidentiality, and decisions to terminate therapy. Cases and codes of ethics are included.

Beauchamp, T., and Walters, L. *Contemporary Issues in Bioethics,* 2nd ed. Belmont, CA: Wadsworth Publishing Co., 1982.

This is an anthology of important essays dealing with such topics as ethical theory, concepts of health and disease, patients' rights and professional responsibilities, abortion, euthanasia, allocation of medical resources, and research.

Benjamin, M., and Curtis, J. *Ethics in Nursing*. New York: Oxford University Press, 1981.

Written by a nurse and a philosopher, this book blends the concrete detail of recurring problems in nursing practice with the perspectives, methods, and resources of philosophical ethics. It stresses the aspects of the nurse's role and relationships with others that make ethical problems in nursing unique. Among the issues addressed are deception, parentalism, confidentiality, conscientious refusal, nurse autonomy, and personal responsibility for institutional and public policy. Several case studies are included in the text and examined in detail; others are grouped in an appendix for analysis by the reader.

Cranford, R. E., and Doudera, A. E., eds. *Institutional Ethics Committees and Health Care Decision Making*. Ann Arbor, MI: Health Administration Press, 1984.

Section 1 consists of the papers, audience discussions, and panel discussions at the first nationwide conference on institutional ethics committees. Sections 2 and 3 include descriptive summaries of extant institutional ethics committees, as well as sample policies and guidelines. This book is a practical resource for those involved in setting up or serving on an institutional ethics committee.

Harron, F., Burnside, J., and Beauchamp, T. *Health and Human Values: A Guide to Making Your Own Decisions*. New Haven: Yale University Press, 1982.

The authors explore such issues as euthanasia, abortion, *in vitro* fertilization, health care and distributive justice, truth telling and informed consent, determination of death and genetic engineering. There are two very practical companion volumes: Shmavonian, N. (compiler). *Human Values in Medicine and Health Care: Audiovisual Resources*. Binghamton, NY: Vale-Ballou Press, 1983. Approximately 400 audiovisual items are listed. Most are annotated and all provide information about purchase and rental. Harron, Frank. *Biomedical and Ethical Issues: A Digest of Law and Policy Development.* Binghamton, NY: Vale-Ballou Press, 1983. This handbook contains excerpts and summaries of influential court decisions, state and federal legislation, and federal guidelines, as well as policy statements from various religious and professional organizations regarding developments in the practice of health care.

Jameton, A. *Nursing Practice: The Ethical Issues.* Englewood Cliffs, NJ: Prentice-Hall, 1984.

This text is a general description and discussion of the clinical and philosophical ethics issues arising in nursing practice. It includes a balanced mixture of cases, methods for resolving nursing ethics problems, and clinical observations, but it is not intended as a clinical handbook, nor does it insist on one particular method for analyzing cases.

Jonsen, A., Seigler, M., and Winslade, W.J. *Clinical Ethics.* New York: Macmillan Co., 1982.

This book examines ethical decision making from a case-based approach. It will be especially helpful for the clinician. Each chapter includes a comprehensive bibliography.

Katz, J. *The Silent World of Doctor and Patient.* New York: Free Press, 1984.

Katz looks at the doctor-patient relationship in order to find the ethical (rather than the legal) basis for informed consent. Although Katz accepts patient autonomy as a primary value, he believes that the physician, because of the ethical obligations of informed consent, has a duty to make sure that the patient's choices are based on a genuine understanding of the way in which treatment decisions will serve the values that the patient actually holds. This view of treatment decisions is based less on patient rights than on decision making as a cooperative activity.

McCormick, R. *Health and Medicine in the Catholic Tradition.* New York: Crossroad Publishing Co., 1984.

This book deals with major questions relating to sexual, medical, and familial morality from the Roman Catholic point of view. Among the issues discussed are birth control and responsible parenthood, abortion, treatment of newborns with disabilities, life-prolonging treatment of the dying, ethical guidelines for the care of the retarded and the aged, and justice in health care.

McCormick, R. *How Brave a New World?* New York: Doubleday, 1981.

One of the foremost Roman Catholic theologians discusses such issues as experimentation, abortion, birth control, reproductive technologies, and the preservation and quality of life. His call for a reevaluation of some traditional Catholic formulations is done with clarity and insight.

O'Rourke, K., and Ashley, B. *Health Care Ethics: A Theological Analysis.* St. Louis: The Catholic Health Association, 1982.

This book explains the traditional Catholic teaching on such things as personhood, the right to health, bioethical decision making, abortion, human experimentation, reproductive technologies, genetic engineering, suffering, and death.

President's Commission for the Study of Ethical Problems in Medicine and Biomedical and Behavioral Research. *Defining Death,* 1981; *Whistleblowing in Biomedical Research,* 1981; *Compensating for Research Injuries,* 2 vols., 1982; *Protecting Human Subjects,* 1981; *Splicing Life,* 1982; *Making Health Care Decisions,* 3 vols., 1982-3; *Deciding to Forego Life-Sustaining Treatment,* 1983; *Implementing Human Research Regulations,* 1983; *Screening and Counselling for Genetic Conditions,* 1983; *Securing Access to Health Care,* 3 vols., 1983; and *Summing Up,* 1983. Washington, DC: U.S. Government Printing Office.

The President's Commission was federally mandated from 1980 to 1983. During its brief life it conducted public hearings across the country and did extensive research on the subjects listed above. The documents produced by the President's Commission are extremely important resources. Each of these is available from the Superintendent of Documents, U.S. Government Printing Office, Washington, DC 20402.

Reich, W. T., ed. *Encyclopedia of Bioethics,* 4 vols. New York: Free Press, 1978.

Four volumes containing excellent basic articles on almost all the issues currently being discussed in biomedical ethics, with references to broader literature in ethics, medicine, and science.

Reiser, S., Dyck, A., and Curran, W. *Ethics in Medicine: Historical Perspectives and Contemporary Concerns.* Cambridge, MA: MIT Press, 1977.

This is one of the most complete anthologies of biomedical ethics available, containing articles on the major issues by philosophers, theologians, physicians, and lawyers. It includes several important historical documents.

Veatch, R. *Case Studies in Medical Ethics.* Cambridge, MA: Harvard University Press, 1977.

In ample supply, the case studies in this book pertain to such topics as health care delivery, duties to patients, confidentiality, truth telling, abortion, genetics, experimentation, and death and dying.

Veatch, R. *Death, Dying, and the Biological Revolution.* New Haven: Yale University Press, 1976.

This book treats the ethical issues surrounding the care of the dying in a careful and comprehensive way. It is generally a good summary of current thinking on these issues.

Veatch, R. *A Theory of Medical Ethics.* New York: Basic Books, 1981.

The author notes that traditional codes of medical ethics are not adequate to the ethical problems in medicine today. He attempts to develop a more comprehensive theory of medical ethics and to apply it to clinical cases.

Weir, R. *Selective Nontreatment of Handicapped Newborns: Moral Dilemmas in Neonatal Medicine.* New York: Oxford University Press, 1984.

This book is the first serious treatment of the ethical dilemmas of neonatal medicine, and it presents a balanced, coherent analysis of the medical, ethical, and legal arguments put forth to date. Numerous case studies highlight the broad range of cases involved.

Winslade, W. J., and Ross, J. W. *Choosing Life or Death: A Guide for Patients, Families, and Health Care Professionals.* New York: Free Press, 1986.

This book uses detailed case studies to discuss the differences in the perspectives of patients, patients' families, physicians, nurses, lawyers, and

policymakers when it comes to making health care decisions. Included are chapters on providing or foregoing treatment for patients with incurable conditions, for seriously ill newborns, and for dialysis patients. In addition, there are chapters on extraordinary forms of reproduction, organ transplantation, experimental treatment, and the problems of health care financing.

Wong, C., and Swazey, J. *Dilemmas of Dying: Policies and Procedures for Decisions Not to Treat.* Boston: G.K. Hall, Medical Publishers, 1981.

The result of a conference, this book explores the medical, moral, legal, and procedural aspects of nontreatment decisions. It is practical and creative.

Newsletters and Journals

American Journal of Law and Medicine (quarterly). American Society of Law and Medicine, 765 Commonwealth Ave., Boston, MA 02215.

Ethical Currents (quarterly). Center for Bioethics, St. Joseph Health System, and the California Association of Catholic Hospitals (CACH), 1121 L St., Ste. 409, Sacramento, CA 95814.

This quarterly is written particularly for members of ethics committees.

Frontlines (quarterly). Center for Applied Biomedical Ethics at Rose Medical Center, 4567 E. Ninth Ave., Denver, CO 80220.

Hastings Center Report (bimonthly). Institute of Society, Ethics, and the Life Sciences, 360 Broadway, Hastings-on-Hudson, NY 10706.

Hospital Ethics (bimonthly). American Hospital Association, 840 N. Lake Shore Dr., Chicago, IL 60611.

Journal of Medicine and Philosophy (quarterly). Society for Health and Human Values, University of Chicago Press, 5801 Ellis Ave., Chicago, IL 60637.

Law, Medicine, and Health Care (bimonthly). American Society of Law and Medicine, 765 Commonwealth Avenue, Boston, MA 02215.

Lineacre Quarterly: A Journal of the Philosophy and Ethics of Medical Practice. National Federation of Catholic Physicians Guilds, 850 Elm Grove Rd., Elm Grove, WI 53122.

Source Bibliographies

BioethicsLine (database). National Library of Medicine Data Base, Medlars Management.

BioethicsLine provides bibliographic information on questions of ethics and public policy arising in health care or biomedical research. Developed at the Center for Bioethics, Kennedy Institute of Ethics, Georgetown University, *BioethicsLine* contains English language citations to material published from 1973 to the present. The database is available through most libraries.

Bibliography of Bioethics (annual). Gale Research Co., Detroit, MI 48226.

This yearly publication contains listings of the material available through *BioethicsLine*.

New Titles in Bioethics (monthly). Center for Bioethics, Kennedy Institute of Ethics, Georgetown University, Washington, DC 20057.

A listing of recent acquisitions by the Bioethics Library at the Kennedy Institute.

Audiovisual Materials

The following list of audiovisual materials is included as a resource for bioethics committees. The materials are listed by format: videocassette/film or filmstrip/slides. Material including study manuals or instructor manuals are noted, if possible.

Videocassettes/16-mm Films

Born Dying. 1983.

This 20-minute film presents the agony of a couple, who suddenly find themselves the parents of a dying baby, and the plight of the neonatal ICU nurse, who must provide care for the infant until a treatment decision is made. The film does not attempt to resolve the treatment/no treatment dilemma; rather it lends structure to the problem by presenting a variety of concerned viewpoints. Instructor/study guide is available. Available as 16mm film for rental or purchase; videocassette ¾ inch, Beta, or VHS for purchase.

Carle Medical Communications
510 W. Main
Urbana, IL 61801
217/384-4838

Code Gray: Ethical Dilemmas in Nursing. 1984.

Code Gray documents four actual situations in which nurses confront ethical dilemmas in their work. The dilemmas focus on the questions of beneficence, autonomy, fidelity, and justice. The 28-minute film offers no easy answers and is designed to trigger discussion among nurses, physicians, and other health workers and consumers. Instructor/study guide is available. Available as 16mm film for rental or purchase; videocassette ¾ inch, Beta, or VHS for purchase.

Fanlight Productions
47 Halifax St.
Boston, MA 02130
617/524-0980

Ethics: It's about Choices. 1984.

This 60-minute video was developed as a tool for ethics committees to use in their development. The production features interviews with national authorities in law, medicine, and philosophy, plus scenarios of experiences taken from the front lines of medicine. The video is accompanied by a workbook. Available as videocassette ¾ inch, VHS, or Beta for purchase or rental.

Romed
4636 E. Ninth Ave.
Denver, CO 80220
303/320-2876

Hard Choices. 1980.

Hard Choices is a six-part series on bioethics produced by KCTS TV in Seattle, WA. Each program from the series presents the ideas and experiences of a variety of scientists, medical doctors, and philosophers. It also includes interviews with patients who have been involved in new medical treatments that have led them to ethical choices beyond presently accepted guidelines. The six one-hour programs include:

- Boy or Girl?
- Genetic Screening
- Human Experiments
- Behavior Control
- Death and Dying
- Doctor, I Want . . . Ethical Dilemmas in Resource Allocation

The series is available as video cassette ¾ inch, Beta, or VHS for purchase or rental.

Carle Medical Communications
510 W. Main
Urbana, IL 61801
217/384-4838

Please Let Me Die. 1974.

This production is the first of two films dealing with the case of Dax Cowart. This 30-minute film takes place 10 months after Cowart was burned over 70 percent of his body, leaving him severely disfigured and blind. At issue is the treatment he continues to receive and his desire to end treatment and die. The focus for the presentation is on conversations between Cowart and psychiatrist Robert White during his hospitalization in the burn unit of the Galveston Medical Center, University of Texas.

Available as videocassette ¾ inch for purchase or rental.

Concern for Dying
250 W. 57th St.
New York, NY 10019
212/246-6962

Dax's Case. 1985

The second film regarding Dax Cowart's case was made almost 10 years after the first. This 60-minute film includes some footage from *Please Let Me Die,* but also presents a retrospective look at the concerns and feelings of Cowart and his family, physician, nurses, and friends as a result of his request that he be allowed to die. Available as 16mm film for rental or purchase; ¾ inch video cassette for purchase.

Concern for Dying
250 West 57th Street
New York, NY 10019
212/246-6962

The Right to Die. 1985.

This film dramatizes the case of a man with ALS who wishes to have his ventilator turned off, fully understanding that it will mean his death. His wife supports the decision, his physician opposes it, and the primary nurse is ambivalent about what is best for the patient. The film presents clearly the ethical and psychological problems faced by health professionals when they are asked to help a competent patient die. Available as 16mm or ¾ inch video cassette for rental or purchase; VHS or Beta II for purchase only.

Carle Medical Communications
510 W. Main St.
Urbana, IL 61801
217/384-4838

Who Should Survive? 1973.

Who Should Survive? is a 26-minute dramatic reenactment of the decision not to treat a Down's syndrome baby with an intestinal blockage at Johns Hopkins Hospital. The case is recreated with the actual doctors and nurses playing their true life roles. Following the dramatization is a multidisciplinary panel discussion of the case. Available as 16mm film for rental or purchase.

Joseph P. Kennedy, Jr. Foundation
Film Service
999 Asylum Ave.
Hartford, CT 06105

Filmstrips/Audiocassettes and Slides/Audiocassettes

Bioethics in Nursing Practice. 1981.

This series presents ethical dilemmas that arise in nursing practice. An introduction to basic ethical principles and values is followed by case examples that demonstrate how dilemmas might be resolved. The series includes:

- Part 1: Accountability in Nursing Practice
- Part 2: Patient Advocacy in Nursing Practice
- Part 3: Human Rights in Nursing Practice
- Part 4: Who Lives, Who Dies, Who Cares?
- Part 5: The Moral Value in Health Care

The series is available as filmstrip/audiocassette (single program or series) and slides/audiocassette (single program or series).

Robert J. Brady & Co.
Bowie, MD 20715
301/262-6300

The Ethical Challenge: Four Biomedical Case Studies. 1975.

This program is designed to be used in a classroom setting to introduce the problems of biomedical ethics. The material presented introduces basic information about scientific advances that raise bioethical issues and then demonstrates these issues through four case studies involving scarce medical resources, behavior control, genetic screening, and when to die. The program includes a detailed teacher's guide with other student activities identified. (Part 1 is 17 minutes; part 2 is 15 minutes.) Available as slide/audiocassette.

Science and Mankind, Inc.
Two Holland Avenue
White Plains, NY 10603

The Ethics of Genetic Control. 1976.

This program is designed to introduce the basic ethical issues that grow out of efforts at genetic control. Part 1 presents a history of genetic control leading up to current technology. Part 2 focuses on society's rights and responsibilities in light of technological advances. Both parts present material through case study format. The program is accompanied by a detailed teacher's guide with other student activities identified. (Part 1 is 19 minutes; Part 2 is 14 minutes.) Available as slide/audiocassette.

Science and Mankind, Inc.
Two Holland Avenue
White Plains, NY 10603

The following sources (in addition to the distributors listed above) have audiovisual materials on bioethics.

Catholic Hospital Association
Books and Audiovisuals Department
4455 Woodson Rd.
St. Louis, MO 63134

Center for Health Care Ethics
St. Louis University School of Medicine
1402 South Grand Blvd.
St. Louis, MO 63104

Concern for Dying
250 West 57th St.
New York, NY 10107

Leaven Press
P.O. Box 40292
Kansas City, MO 64141

Society for Health and Human Values
Suite 3A
1311A Dolley Madison Blvd.
McLean, VA 22101

University of California at Los Angeles
Instructional Media Library
Royce Hall, Room 8
405 Hilgard Ave.
Los Angeles, CA 90024

WGBU-TV
Bowling Green State University
Bowling Green, OH 43403

Index